PREGNANCY BONE HEALTH COOKBOOK

A Comprehensive Guide to Osteoporosis Prevention and Bone Health Nutrition for Expectant and New Mothers

DREW DORSEY

Copyright © 2024 by DRE DORSEY

content

Prenatal Vitamins and Bone Health: 77

Managing Osteoporosis Risk Factors   79

Preparing for Postpartum Bone Health   81

Conclusion 85

WELCOME! BUILD STRONG BONES, NOURISH MOM & BABY.

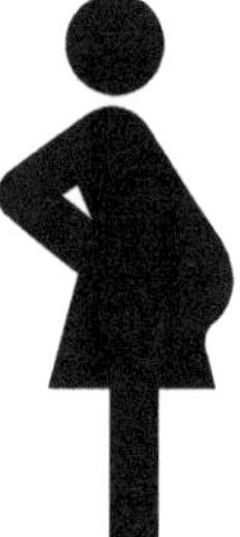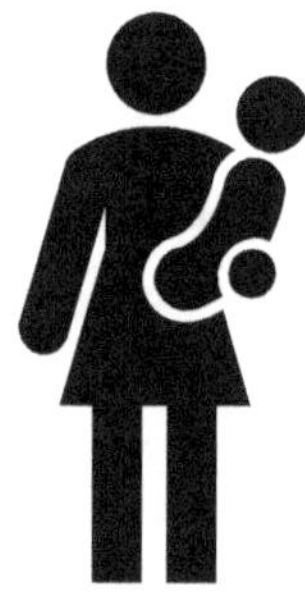

Step into the extraordinary realm of pregnancy where resilience intertwines with delectable flavors!

Congratulations! You're about to embark on the exhilarating voyage of pregnancy. Amidst the bubbling excitement and joyful anticipation, concerns about bone health might be gently nudging your thoughts. Fear not, dear mama-to-be! This cookbook is not merely a collection of recipes; it's your steadfast companion on a journey to fortify a robust foundation – for both you and your precious bundle of joy.

Did you know that pregnancy can be a litmus test for your bones? As your little one grows, it siphons calcium from your bones to fuel its own development. This delicate balance can lead to bone depletion unless your body receives a steady supply of vital nutrients. But worry not! You wield an extraordinary power to safeguard your bone health throughout pregnancy, and this cookbook is your covert arsenal.

Picture this...

A surge of confidence and empowerment as you nourish yourself and your growing baby with the finest sustenance.

Indulging in sumptuous, gratifying dishes that not only tantalize your taste buds but also fortify your bones.

Unearthing straightforward, yet potent strategies to navigate the labyrinth of bone health during this transformative journey.

Acquiring invaluable insights into essential nutrients and their pivotal role in crafting resilient bones for you and your little one.

This cookbook unveils the blueprint for a pregnancy journey anchored in strength. Within its pages, you'll unearth a treasury of mouthwatering recipes meticulously curated with bone-nourishing elements in mind. Whether you're a kitchen virtuoso or a novice culinary adventurer, these recipes are tailored to be:

Effortless to whip up: With straightforward instructions and easily accessible ingredients, you can conjure up wholesome meals even amidst the hustle and bustle of life.

Overflowing with flavor and satiation: Bid farewell to uninspiring, health-centric meals! These culinary creations burst with taste, satisfying your cravings, and fueling your vitality.

Adaptable and versatile: Dietary constraints? Consider them conquered! Many recipes offer variations to accommodate diverse needs and preferences.

From sunrise breakfasts to moonlit suppers and every nibble in between, this cookbook leaves no culinary stone unturned. We'll walk you through integrating bone-building powerhouses like dairy, verdant greens, succulent fruits, hearty grains, and protein-rich delights into your daily fare. But our journey doesn't stop at the kitchen stove. You'll also unearth invaluable insights and advice on:

- Deciphering the intricacies of osteoporosis and its resonance during pregnancy.
- Optimizing nutrient absorption to foster peak bone health.
- Cultivating a wholesome lifestyle through mindful choices and invigorating exercise.
- Fostering the confidence to make informed decisions throughout your pregnancy odyssey.

Pregnancy is an enchanting saga of marvel and metamorphosis. Allow this cookbook to be your steadfast ally on this enchanting journey. Together, we'll nourish your body, fortify your bones, and forge a robust foundation for a radiant pregnancy and a flourishing future for you and your precious little one.

Understanding Osteoporosis and Pregnancy can be a complex journey for expectant mothers, filled with both anticipation and concern. Osteoporosis, often dubbed the "silent disease," silently weakens bones over time, making them fragile and susceptible to fractures. For pregnant women, the prospect of managing this condition alongside the joys and challenges of pregnancy can evoke a whirlwind of emotions.

Imagine the anxiety a pregnant woman might feel upon learning that she has osteoporosis or is at risk for it. ***Questions flood her mind:*** *How will this affect my baby? Can I still have a healthy pregnancy? What precautions do I need to take?*

Osteoporosis doesn't pause during pregnancy; if anything, the stakes feel higher. Pregnancy places additional strain on a woman's body, as it works overtime to nourish and support the growing life within. The hormonal changes that accompany pregnancy can further impact bone health, making it essential for expectant mothers to understand the intricacies of this condition. As she delves deeper into understanding osteoporosis and pregnancy, she learns about the importance of bone density and strength for both her and her baby. She discovers that while pregnancy-related hormonal shifts may temporarily increase bone turnover, her body is designed to adapt and prioritize the needs of her growing child. Yet, she also learns that women with pre-existing osteoporosis face heightened risks of fractures and other complications during pregnancy and childbirth.

With this knowledge comes empowerment. Armed with information and supported by healthcare providers who specialize in maternal-fetal medicine and bone health, she navigates her pregnancy journey with confidence. She learns to balance the need for adequate nutrition, safe exercise, and regular prenatal care to optimize both her bone health and the health of her baby. Understanding osteoporosis and pregnancy isn't just about facts and figures; it's about embracing vulnerability and strength in equal measure. It's about acknowledging the challenges while finding resilience in the face of uncertainty. Ultimately, it's about embarking on a journey of motherhood with courage, determination, and a deep-rooted commitment to nurturing both body and soul.

Importance of Bone Health during Pregnancy

During pregnancy, bone health often takes a backseat to the immediate concerns of childbirth and prenatal care. However, the significance of maintaining strong and healthy bones during this transformative time cannot be overstated. As a mother-to-be, nurturing your bone health is not just about ensuring your own well-being, but also laying the foundation for the healthy development of your baby.

Imagine the intricate dance of nutrients and minerals within your body, each playing a crucial role in supporting the growth and development of your unborn child. Calcium, often referred to as the building block of bones, takes center stage during pregnancy. Your growing baby relies on a steady supply of calcium to form their own skeletal structure, ensuring that they enter the world with a solid foundation for a healthy life.

But here's the twist: your baby isn't the only one drawing from your calcium reserves. As your pregnancy progresses, your body undergoes a myriad of changes, including hormonal shifts that can affect your bone density. Without adequate calcium intake, your body may begin to leach calcium from your bones to meet the demands of your growing baby, putting you at risk of osteoporosis and fractures later in life.

Furthermore, the strains and stresses of pregnancy, coupled with the physical demands of childbirth, can exacerbate existing bone health issues or create new ones altogether. From the aches and pains of carrying extra weight to the hormonal fluctuations that accompany breastfeeding, your bones endure a remarkable journey alongside you.

That's why prioritizing bone health during pregnancy isn't just about preventing fractures or osteoporosis in the distant future—it's about safeguarding your vitality and resilience as a mother. By nourishing your body with calcium-rich foods, engaging in safe exercises that promote bone strength, and seeking guidance from healthcare providers, you can empower yourself to embrace the challenges of pregnancy with confidence and grace, knowing that you're investing in a future filled with joy, laughter, and boundless possibilities—for both you and your baby.

What is Osteoporosis?

Osteoporosis is a disorder that impairs bone density and strength. Consider your bones to be brick-built structures. In osteoporosis, the bricks (which are the minerals like calcium and phosphate in your bones) become weaker and more fragile. This weakening increases your risk of fractures, even from minor falls or bumps that wouldn't normally cause harm.

Now, you might be wondering how this happens. Well, normally, your body is constantly breaking down old bone tissue and replacing it with new bone. But in osteoporosis, this balance is disrupted. Your body either breaks down bone too quickly, doesn't make enough new bone, or both. As a result, your bones become thinner and less dense over time.

Osteoporosis often doesn't cause any symptoms in the early stages, which is why it's sometimes called a "silent disease." But as it progresses, you might notice symptoms like back pain, loss of height, and a stooped posture. These can be signs that your bones are becoming weak and prone to fractures.

Diagnosing osteoporosis typically involves a bone density test called a DEXA scan. This painless procedure measures the mineral content in your bones and helps determine your risk of fractures.

The good news is that osteoporosis can be managed and treated, especially if detected early.

Treatment may include lifestyle changes like regular exercise and a healthy diet rich in calcium

and vitamin D, as well as medications to strengthen bones and reduce fracture risk.

Causes and Risk Factors of Osteoporosis:

Age: As we age, our bones naturally lose density, becoming weaker and more prone to

fractures. Osteoporosis is more common in older adults, particularly in women after menopause.

Hormonal Changes: Estrogen is important for maintaining bone density. After menopause,

when estrogen levels decline, women are at increased risk of osteoporosis. Similarly, hormonal

disorders or treatments that disrupt hormone levels can also contribute to bone loss.

Nutritional Deficiencies: Inadequate intake of calcium and vitamin D, essential nutrients

for bone health, can increase the risk of osteoporosis. Additionally, certain medical conditions or

medications may interfere with the absorption or utilization of these nutrients.

Family History: If you have a family member with osteoporosis, you may be genetically

predisposed to the condition. Genetic factors can influence bone density and structure, affecting

your risk of developing osteoporosis.

<u>Lifestyle Factors:</u> Certain lifestyle habits can contribute to bone loss and increase the risk of osteoporosis. These include smoking, excessive alcohol consumption, sedentary behavior, and a diet low in calcium and vitamin D.

<u>Medical Conditions:</u> Chronic conditions such as rheumatoid arthritis, celiac disease, and inflammatory bowel disease can impact bone health and increase the risk of osteoporosis. Similarly, long-term use of corticosteroid medications can weaken bones over time.

Impact on Pregnancy and Postpartum Health:

Osteoporosis during pregnancy and postpartum presents unique challenges and considerations for both the mother and her baby. Pregnancy itself can accelerate bone loss, particularly in women who already have low bone density or other risk factors for osteoporosis. Hormonal changes, increased calcium demands from the developing fetus, and changes in physical activity levels during pregnancy can further exacerbate bone loss.

Moreover, fractures during pregnancy and childbirth can have serious consequences for both maternal and fetal health. Fractures can complicate delivery and increase the risk of complications such as excessive bleeding or prolonged labor. Postpartum, fractures can impair mobility and hinder the mother's ability to care for herself and her newborn.

In addition to the immediate concerns during pregnancy and childbirth, osteoporosis can have long-term implications for postpartum health. Women with osteoporosis are at increased risk of fractures, which can impact their quality of life, independence, and ability to care for their children.

How This Book Can Help:

This book aims to provide comprehensive guidance and support for pregnant women facing osteoporosis or concerned about their bone health during and after pregnancy. By addressing the causes, risk factors, and potential impact of osteoporosis on pregnancy and postpartum health, this book empowers women to take proactive steps to manage the condition and reduce their risk of fractures. Through evidence-based advice, practical tips, and personalized strategies, readers can gain the knowledge and confidence to prioritize their bone health and navigate the challenges of pregnancy and motherhood with resilience and vitality.

macronutrients and Micronutrients for Bone Health

Absolutely, let's break down the relevance of macronutrients and micronutrients for bone health in an understandable manner.

When we talk about bone health, it's not just about drinking milk for calcium. Our bones are complex structures that require a variety of nutrients to stay strong and resilient. Think of it like building a sturdy house – you need more than just bricks; you need a solid foundation, too.

Macronutrients:

Protein: Protein is like the building blocks of our body, including our bones. It's essential for bone growth, repair, and maintenance. Without enough protein, our bones can become weak and brittle. Lean meats, poultry, fish, eggs, dairy products, legumes, nuts, and seeds are all excellent sources of protein.

Fats: Healthy fats play a role in absorbing fat-soluble vitamins like vitamin D, which is crucial for calcium absorption and bone health. Omega-3 fatty acids, found in fatty fish, flaxseeds, chia seeds, and walnuts, have anti-inflammatory properties that can help reduce bone loss and improve bone density.

Carbohydrates: Carbohydrates provide energy for our bodies, including the energy needed for bone remodeling – the process of breaking down and rebuilding bone tissue. opt for complex carbohydrates like whole grains, fruits, vegetables, and legumes, which also provide important vitamins and minerals for bone health.

Micronutrients:

Calcium: Calcium is the superstar nutrient when it comes to bone health. It's the main mineral found in our bones and teeth, giving them strength and structure. Dairy products like milk, yogurt, and cheese are well-known sources of calcium, but you can also find it in leafy greens, tofu, almonds, and fortified foods.

Vitamin D: The body needs vitamin D in order to absorb calcium. Without enough vitamin D, your body can't effectively use the calcium you consume, leading to weakened bones. Get your daily dose of vitamin D from sunlight exposure (about 10-30 minutes a few times a week), fatty fish, fortified foods like milk and orange juice, and supplements if necessary.

Vitamin K: Vitamin K helps regulate calcium in the body and is involved in bone mineralization – the process of turning calcium into bone tissue. Leafy greens like spinach, kale, and broccoli are excellent sources of vitamin K, along with fermented foods like sauerkraut and natto.

By ensuring you get the right balance of macronutrients and micronutrients through a varied and balanced diet, you're giving your bones the nutrients they need to stay strong and healthy for years to come. Think of it as nourishing your bones from the inside out, so they can continue to support you in all your daily activities, whether it's walking, running, or simply carrying groceries.

Think of your body as a complex machine that needs the right fuel to function properly. During pregnancy, your body has increased demands for certain nutrients to support both your own health and the growth of your baby. ***Two key nutrients for bone health are calcium and vitamin D.***

- ❖ For calcium, the recommended daily intake during pregnancy is around 1,000 milligrams per day. This is crucial for building your baby's bones and teeth, as well as maintaining your own bone density. Good sources of calcium include dairy products like milk, yogurt, and cheese, as well as leafy green vegetables like spinach and kale, and fortified foods like tofu and orange juice.

- ❖ Vitamin D is also essential for calcium absorption and bone health. Your body can produce vitamin D when your skin is exposed to sunlight, but during pregnancy, you may need additional sources to meet your needs. The recommended daily intake for vitamin D during pregnancy is around 600 international units (IU) per day. Good food sources of vitamin D include fatty fish like salmon and tuna, fortified dairy and plant-based milk, eggs, and mushrooms.

Sources of Other Vital Nutrients, Vitamin D, and Calcium:

Now, let's talk about where you can find these nutrients in your everyday diet. Incorporating a variety of foods rich in calcium and vitamin D can help ensure you're meeting your daily needs.

❖ For calcium, try to include dairy products like milk, yogurt, and cheese in your meals and snacks. If you're lactose intolerant or prefer plant-based options, you can also choose fortified dairy alternatives like almond milk or soy milk, as well as calcium-fortified foods like tofu, cereals, and orange juice. Leafy green vegetables such as broccoli, kale, and collard greens are also excellent sources of calcium.

❖ As for vitamin D, aim to include fatty fish like salmon, mackerel, and sardines in your diet regularly. Eggs, fortified dairy products, and fortified cereals are also good sources. And don't forget about sunlight! Spending some time outdoors each day can help your body produce vitamin D naturally.

In addition to calcium and vitamin D, it's important to maintain a balanced diet rich in other essential nutrients like protein, iron, and folate. Lean meats, poultry, beans, lentils, nuts, seeds, whole grains, fruits, and vegetables are all important components of a healthy pregnancy diet.

How Pregnancy Affects Bone Density

During pregnancy, your body undergoes a series of remarkable changes to support the growth and development of your baby. Hormones, nutrition, and physiological adaptations interact delicately to orchestrate these changes. While pregnancy is often celebrated as a time of joy and anticipation, it's important to recognize that it can also have implications for your bone health. One of the key hormones involved in pregnancy is estrogen. Estrogen plays a crucial role in maintaining bone density by inhibiting the activity of cells called osteoclasts, which are responsible for breaking down bone tissue. However, during pregnancy, estrogen levels rise significantly, reaching their peak in the third trimester. This surge in estrogen can lead to a temporary suppression of bone turnover, resulting in a slight increase in bone density.

<u>But here's the catch:</u> while estrogen levels are elevated during pregnancy, so too are the demands on your body for calcium and other nutrients to support the growth of your baby's bones and teeth. Your baby relies on a steady supply of calcium from your bones to fuel their own skeletal development. As a result, some studies suggest that pregnancy can actually lead to a small loss of bone density in certain areas of the skeleton, particularly the spine and hip. Furthermore, the physical demands of pregnancy, such as the increased weight of the growing uterus and changes in posture, can place additional stress on your bones and joints. This can contribute to discomfort, aches, and pains, particularly in areas like the lower back and pelvis. After childbirth, the hormonal landscape of your body undergoes yet another shift. Estrogen levels plummet, sometimes reaching levels even lower than those experienced during menopause. This rapid decline in estrogen can trigger an acceleration of bone turnover, leading to a temporary loss of bone density known as postpartum bone loss.

Fortunately, for most women, this bone loss is transient and reversible. In the months following childbirth, as hormone levels stabilize and breastfeeding ceases, your body gradually rebuilds lost bone tissue. However, for women with pre-existing risk factors for osteoporosis or those who experience prolonged breastfeeding, the postpartum period may represent a critical window of vulnerability for bone health.

Pregnancy can have complex and multifaceted effects on bone density. While the temporary changes in bone turnover and density during pregnancy and postpartum are generally considered normal physiological adaptations, it's important to prioritize bone health through adequate nutrition, weight-bearing exercise, and regular prenatal care. If you have concerns about your bone health during pregnancy or postpartum, don't hesitate to discuss them with your healthcare provider. By working together, you can develop a personalized plan to support your bone health and ensure a healthy pregnancy and postpartum recovery.

Risks and Complications for Women with Osteoporosis:

Pregnancy presents unique challenges for women with osteoporosis, as the physiological changes and hormonal fluctuations can exacerbate existing bone health issues. Women with osteoporosis are at increased risk of fractures during pregnancy and childbirth, which can lead to complications for both the mother and her baby.

Fractures during pregnancy can cause pain, mobility limitations, and discomfort, making it more challenging for women to navigate the physical demands of pregnancy. In severe cases, fractures may require medical intervention or even surgical repair, which can further complicate prenatal care and delivery.

Moreover, fractures during pregnancy can impact the birthing process itself. Fractures of the pelvis or spine can interfere with the baby's descent through the birth canal, potentially necessitating interventions such as cesarean section delivery. Fractures can also increase the risk of complications during labor and delivery, such as excessive bleeding or prolonged labor. Beyond the immediate concerns during pregnancy and childbirth, osteoporosis can have long-term implications for postpartum health. Women with osteoporosis are at increased risk of fractures during the postpartum period, particularly if they breastfeed, as breastfeeding can further deplete calcium stores in the body.

Preventive Measures During Pregnancy:

While pregnancy poses unique challenges for women with osteoporosis, there are several preventive measures that can help minimize the risks and complications associated with the condition:

Nutritional Support: Ensuring adequate intake of calcium and vitamin D is crucial for maintaining bone health during pregnancy. Women with osteoporosis may require higher doses of these nutrients to meet their increased needs. A balanced diet rich in calcium-rich foods like dairy products, leafy greens, and fortified foods, coupled with vitamin D supplementation, if necessary, can help support bone health during pregnancy.

Weight-Bearing Exercise: Engaging in regular, low-impact exercises such as walking, swimming, or prenatal yoga can help strengthen bones and improve overall bone density. However, it's important to consult with a healthcare provider before starting any new exercise regimen, especially if you have osteoporosis or other medical conditions.

Fall Prevention: Taking precautions to minimize the risk of falls can help prevent fractures during pregnancy. This may include wearing supportive footwear, using handrails on stairs, and avoiding activities that increase the risk of falls, such as high-impact sports or activities with uneven terrain.

<u>Medication Management:</u> Women with severe osteoporosis or those at high risk of fractures may require medication to help manage the condition during pregnancy. However, it's essential to discuss the risks and benefits of any medications with a healthcare provider, as some medications may not be safe during pregnancy or breastfeeding.

<u>Regular Prenatal Care:</u> Maintaining regular prenatal care appointments allows healthcare providers to monitor your bone health and address any concerns or complications that may arise. Your healthcare team can provide personalized guidance and support to help manage osteoporosis during pregnancy and ensure the best possible outcomes for you and your baby.

By taking proactive steps to support bone health during pregnancy, women with osteoporosis can minimize the risks and complications associated with the condition and enjoy a healthy pregnancy and postpartum recovery. If you have osteoporosis and are planning a pregnancy or are already pregnant, be sure to discuss your concerns with your healthcare provider. Together, you can develop a personalized plan to optimize your bone health and ensure a safe and healthy pregnancy journey.

Importance of Exercise for Bone Strength:

Stimulates Bone Formation: Weight-bearing exercises such as walking, jogging, dancing, and strength training stimulate the bones to build new tissue, increasing bone density and strength over time. Just as muscles grow stronger with exercise, bones respond to the stress placed on them by becoming denser and more resilient.

Helps Maintain Bone Mass: As we age, our bodies naturally lose bone mass, leading to conditions like osteopenia and osteoporosis. Regular exercise, particularly weight-bearing and resistance exercises, can help slow down this loss of bone mass and reduce the risk of fractures and osteoporosis-related complications.

Improves Balance and Coordination: Balance and coordination exercises, such as yoga, tai chi, and Pilates, can help improve stability and reduce the risk of falls, which are a major cause of fractures, especially in older adults. By strengthening the muscles around the joints and improving proprioception (awareness of body position), these exercises can help prevent accidents and injuries.

Enhances Joint Health: Exercise helps keep the joints flexible and lubricated, reducing the risk of stiffness, pain, and inflammation associated with conditions like osteoarthritis. By promoting joint mobility and function, exercise can improve overall musculoskeletal health and quality of life.

Promotes Overall Health and Well-being: Regular physical activity has numerous benefits beyond bone health, including cardiovascular fitness, weight management, stress reduction, and mood enhancement. By incorporating exercise into your daily routine, you can improve your overall health and well-being, reducing the risk of chronic diseases and promoting longevity.

Can Be Adapted to Individual Needs: Exercise is highly versatile and can be tailored to individual preferences, fitness levels, and physical abilities. Whether you prefer walking, swimming, cycling, or strength training, there are plenty of options to choose from. Even small amounts of exercise can make a big difference in bone health, so finding activities that you enjoy and can stick with is key.

<u>**Provides Social Interaction:**</u> Many forms of exercise, such as group fitness classes, team sports, or walking clubs, offer opportunities for social interaction and camaraderie. Building connections with others who share similar health and fitness goals can provide motivation and support, making it easier to stay active and maintain a consistent exercise routine.

Overall, exercise is a critical component of maintaining strong and healthy bones throughout life. By incorporating regular physical activity into your lifestyle, you can strengthen your bones, improve your overall health, and enjoy a more active and fulfilling life. If you're unsure where to start or have concerns about exercising safely, consider consulting with a healthcare provider or certified fitness professional for personalized guidance and support.

Safe and Effective Exercises for Pregnant Women

<u>**Walking:**</u> Walking is one of the safest and easiest forms of exercise for pregnant women. It's low-impact, gentle on the joints, and can be done almost anywhere, making it an ideal choice for all fitness levels. Every day of the week, try to get in at least 30 minutes of brisk walking to enhance circulation and gain the advantages of cardiovascular fitness.

<u>**Swimming and Water Aerobics:**</u> Swimming and water aerobics are excellent options for pregnant women, as the buoyancy of water reduces stress on the joints and provides gentle resistance for muscle strengthening. Water exercises can help improve cardiovascular fitness, promote flexibility, and relieve discomfort associated with pregnancy-related swelling and back pain.

Prenatal Yoga: Prenatal yoga focuses on gentle stretching, breathing techniques, and relaxation exercises specifically tailored to the needs of pregnant women. Yoga can help improve flexibility, balance, and posture, while also promoting relaxation and stress reduction. Seek out prenatal yoga courses or instructional DVDs taught by qualified teachers who understand how to adjust poses during pregnancy.

<u>**Pilates:**</u> Pilates is a low-impact exercise method that focuses on strengthening the core muscles, pelvic floor, and postural muscles. Prenatal Pilates classes typically emphasize safe and effective exercises for pregnant women, helping to improve posture, stability, and muscle tone. Be sure to choose a certified instructor with experience in prenatal Pilates.

<u>**Stationary Cycling:**</u> Stationary cycling or indoor cycling classes are safe options for pregnant women, as they provide a low-impact cardiovascular workout without the risk of falls or injury.

Adjust the resistance and intensity to your comfort level and avoid standing or high-intensity intervals that could strain the pelvic floor muscles.

Strength Training with Lightweight Weights: During pregnancy, strength training routines with small weights or resistance bands can help preserve muscular tone and strength. Concentrate on workouts like bicep curls, shoulder presses, squats, and lunges that target large muscle groups. Avoid heavy lifting, especially exercises that require lying on your back or putting excessive strain on the abdominal muscles.

<u>Pelvic Floor Exercises (Kegels):</u> Pelvic floor exercises, also known as Kegels, are essential for maintaining pelvic floor strength and preventing urinary incontinence during and after pregnancy. To perform Kegels, contract the muscles of the pelvic floor as if you were stopping the flow of urine, hold for a few seconds, then release. Aim for 10-15 repetitions, several times a day.

It's important to listen to your body and modify exercises as needed to accommodate changes in balance, flexibility, and comfort during pregnancy. Always consult with your healthcare provider before starting any new exercise program, especially if you have any underlying medical conditions or pregnancy complications. If you experience any pain, dizziness, or discomfort while exercising, stop immediately and seek medical advice.

lifestyle factors that can impact bone health.

Our bones are living tissues that respond to the environment we create for them through our lifestyle choices. Several lifestyle factors play a significant role in determining bone health and density, influencing our risk of conditions like osteoporosis and fractures.

Dietary Habits: A balanced diet rich in calcium, vitamin D, and other essential nutrients is crucial for maintaining strong and healthy bones. Inadequate intake of calcium and vitamin D can weaken bones over time, increasing the risk of fractures and osteoporosis. On the other hand, a diet high in processed foods, excessive sodium, and sugary beverages can have detrimental effects on bone health.

Physical Activity Levels: Regular exercise, particularly weight-bearing and resistance exercises, is essential for building and maintaining bone density. Sedentary lifestyles, on the other hand, can lead to bone loss and decreased muscle strength, increasing the risk of falls and fractures, especially as we age.

Smoking: Smoking has been linked to decreased bone density and an increased risk of fractures, particularly in postmenopausal women. Smoking interferes with the absorption of calcium and other nutrients, reduces estrogen levels, and impairs bone formation and repair processes.

Alcohol Consumption: Excessive alcohol consumption can interfere with bone remodeling and increase the risk of osteoporosis and fractures. Alcohol abuse can disrupt the balance of hormones involved in bone metabolism and impair the body's ability to absorb calcium and other essential nutrients.

Body Weight and Composition: Maintaining a healthy body weight and body composition is important for bone health. Both obesity and underweight can negatively impact bone density and increase the risk of fractures. Excess body fat can produce inflammatory cytokines that promote bone resorption, while low body weight can lead to hormonal imbalances that affect bone metabolism.

By adopting healthy lifestyle habits, such as eating a balanced diet, staying physically active, avoiding smoking and excessive alcohol consumption, and maintaining a healthy weight, we can support optimal bone health and reduce the risk of fractures and osteoporosis as we age. Making small, sustainable changes to our daily routines can have a significant impact on our long-term bone health and overall well-being.

Building a Bone-Friendly Diet Plan

Calcium

Dairy products: Milk, cheese, yogurt

Dark leafy vegetables (except spinach): Kale, collard greens, mustard greens

Fortified foods: Cereals, orange juice

Sardines

Tofu

Vitamin D

Fatty fish: Salmon, tuna, mackerel

Egg yolks

Beef liver.

Mushrooms (when exposed to UV light)

Fortified foods: Milk, cereals, yogurt

Magnesium

Green leafy vegetables: Spinach, kale, Swiss chard

Nuts and seeds: Almonds, cashews, pumpkin seeds

Whole grains: Brown rice, quinoa, oats

Legumes: Beans, lentils, chickpeas

Phosphorus

Dairy products: Milk, cheese, yogurt

Meat, poultry, and fish

Eggs

Whole grains

Beans and lentils

Vitamin K

Leafy green veggies include kale, spinach, collard greens, and Swiss chard.

Natto (fermented soybean dish)

Protein

Lean meats: Chicken, turkey, fish

Eggs

Beans and lentils

Tofu

Nuts and seeds.

Vitamin C

Citrus fruits: Oranges, grapefruits, lemons, limes

Berries: Strawberries, blueberries, raspberries

Bell peppers

Tomatoes

Potassium

Fruits: Bananas, cantaloupe, oranges, honeydew melon

Vegetables: Potatoes, sweet potatoes, spinach, tomatoes

Beans and lentils

Manganese

Nuts and seeds: Almonds, cashews, walnuts, pecans.

Whole grains: Brown rice, quinoa, oats

Legumes: Beans, lentils, chickpeas

Leafy green vegetables: Spinach, kale, collard greens

Pineapple

Copper

Shellfish: Oysters, clams, crabs, lobsters

Organ meats: Liver, kidney

Nuts and seeds: Cashews, almonds, sunflower seeds

Whole grains: Quinoa, whole-wheat bread

Dark chocolate

Boron

Nuts and seeds: Almonds, peanuts, raisins.

Prunes

Avocados

Apples

Pears

Iron

Lean meats: Beef, lamb, pork

Poultry: Chicken, turkey

Fish: Tuna, sardines, salmon

Beans and lentils

Dark leafy green vegetables: Spinach, kale

Zinc

Oysters

Red meat

Poultry

Beans and lentils

Nuts and seeds.

Vitamin A

Orange and yellow veggies include carrots, sweet potatoes, and butternut squash.

Dark leafy green vegetables: Kale, spinach, collard greens

Fatty fish: Salmon, tuna, and mackerel

Liver

Milk and dairy products.

Breakfast recipes.

High-Protein Yogurt Bowl

Ingredients:

- 1 cup Greek yogurt (plain or flavored)
- ½ cup berries (fresh or frozen)
- ¼ cup sliced almonds
- 2 tablespoons granola (fortified)

Preparation Method:

- In a bowl, layer the Greek yogurt.
- Top with berries, sliced almonds, and granola.

Instructions:

- No cooking is required. Simply assemble the ingredients in the bowl.

Total Preparation Time: 5 minutes

Serving Size: 1 bowl

Nutritional Value (approximate):
Calories: 350-400
Protein: 20-25 grams
Carbohydrates: 40-50 grams
Fat: 10-15 grams
Calcium: 200-300mg (depending on yogurt)
Vitamin D: (fortified yogurt)

Scrambled Eggs with Kale and Cheese

Ingredients:

- 2 eggs

- ➢ 1 cup chopped kale.
- ➢ ¼ cup shredded cheese
- ➢ 1 tablespoon butter or olive oil
- ➢ Salt and pepper to taste

Preparation Method:

- • Wash and chop the kale.
- • In a pan, heat the butter or olive oil over medium heat.
- • Add the chopped kale and cook until slightly wilted, about 2 minutes.

Instructions:

- • Whisk the eggs in a bowl with a splash of water or milk.
- • Season with salt and pepper.
- • Pour the egg mixture into the pan with the kale.
- • Scramble the eggs until cooked through, about 3-5 minutes.
- • Sprinkle the shredded cheese over the cooked eggs and let it melt for a few seconds.

Cooking Time: 5 minutes

Total Preparation Time: 10 minutes

Serving Size: 1 serving

Nutritional Value (approximate):
Calories: 250-300
Protein: 15-20 grams
Carbohydrates: 2-3 grams
Fat: 15-20 grams
Calcium: (from cheese)
Vitamin D: (from eggs)

Tofu Scramble with Bell Peppers

Ingredients:

- ➢ One block (14 ounces) of firm tofu, drained and pressed.
- ➢ 1 tablespoon olive oil

> ½ cup chopped bell peppers (any color)

> ¼ cup chopped onion (optional)

> ½ teaspoon turmeric powder

> Salt and pepper to taste

> ¼ cup chopped fresh parsley (optional)

> Side of roasted sweet potato (optional)

Preparation Method:

- Use your hands or a fork to crumble the tofu.

- Chop the bell peppers and onion (if using).

Instructions:

- In a pan, heat the olive oil over medium heat.

- Add the chopped onion (if using) and cook until softened, about 2 minutes.

- Add the diced bell peppers and simmer for another 2-3 minutes.

- Add the crumbled tofu and turmeric powder.

- Sauté for 5-7 minutes, breaking up the tofu further with a spatula.

- Season with salt and pepper to taste.

- Garnish with chopped fresh parsley (if using).

Cooking Time:10 minutes

Total Preparation Time: 15 minutes (including roasting sweet potato, if using)

Serving Size: 1 serving

Nutritional Value (approximate):
Calories: 300-350
Protein: 20-25 grams
Carbohydrates: 20-25 grams (depending on sweet potato)
Fat: 10-15 grams
Calcium: (from fortified plant-based milk, if used)

<u>**Fortified Cereal with Milk and Fruit**</u>

Ingredients:

- 1 cup fortified cereal
- 1 cup low-fat milk
- ½ cup chopped fruit (fresh or frozen)

Preparation Method:

- Wash and chop the fruit (if using fresh).

Instructions:

- Pour the cereal into a bowl.
- Add milk and stir to combine.
- Top with chopped fruit.

Total Preparation Time: 2 minutes

Serving Size: 1 bowl

Nutritional Value (approximate):
Calories: 250-300
Protein: 10-15 grams
Carbohydrates: 30–40 grams
Fat: 5–10 grams
Calcium: (from milk)
Vitamin D:

<u>**Salmon and Veggie Frittata**</u>

Ingredients:

- 4 eggs
- 1/4 cup milk (dairy or fortified)
- 1/4 cup chopped kale or spinach.
- 1/2 cup chopped cooked salmon (flaked)
- 1/4 cup chopped red bell pepper.
- 1/4 cup chopped onion.
- 1 tablespoon olive oil

> ➢ Salt and pepper to taste

> ➢ 1/4 cup shredded cheese (optional)

Preparation Method:

- Preheat oven to 400°F (200°C). Grease a ten-inch oven-safe skillet or pie plate.

- In a large bowl, whisk together eggs and milk. Season with salt and pepper.

- Heat olive oil in the skillet over medium heat. Add onions and cook until softened, about 3 minutes.

- Add chopped bell peppers and kale/spinach. Sauté for a further two to three minutes, or until wilted.

- Remove vegetables from the pan and set aside.

- Pour the egg mixture into the preheated skillet. Stir in the cooked vegetables and flaked salmon.

- Sprinkle with shredded cheese (optional).

- Bake for 20-25 minutes, or until the center is set and a toothpick inserted comes out clean.

- Let cool slightly before slicing and serving.

Cooking Time: 20-25 minutes

Total Preparation Time: 30 minutes

Serving Size: 4 wedges

Nutrition Value (per serving):
Calories: Around 300 (depending on ingredients)
Protein: Around 20g
Fat: Around 15g
Carbohydrates: Around 10g
Calcium: Around 100mg (depending on cheese)
Vitamin D: Small amount from eggs

Nut Butter and Banana Smoothie

Ingredients:

- ➢ 1 cup milk (dairy or fortified)
- ➢ 1/2 cup plain yogurt (Greek yogurt recommended for extra protein)
- ➢ 1 ripe banana
- ➢ 2 tablespoons nut butter (peanut butter, almond butter, etc.)
- ➢ 1/2 teaspoon ground cinnamon (optional)
- ➢ 1/4 cup ice cubes (optional)

Preparation Method:

- In a blender, combine all ingredients and process until smooth and creamy.

Cooking Time: N/A (blending only)

Total Preparation Time: 5 minutes

Serving Size: 1 person

Nutrition Value (per serving, using peanut butter):
Calories: Around 300
Protein: Around 20g
Fat: Around 10g
Carbohydrates: Around 40g
Calcium: Around 300mg (depending on yogurt)
Vitamin D: Small amount from milk (if fortified)

Turkey Sausage and Whole-Wheat Toast

Ingredients:

- ➢ 2 turkey sausage links
- ➢ 2 slices whole-wheat bread
- ➢ 1 tablespoon butter or olive oil
- ➢ 1 sliced tomato (optional)
- ➢ Salt and pepper to taste

Preparation Method:

- Put some oil or butter in a pan and heat it to medium.
- Cook turkey sausage links according to package instructions, turning occasionally.

- Meanwhile, toast whole-wheat bread slices to desired doneness.

- Place sausage links on toasted bread.

- Top with sliced tomato (optional) and season with salt and pepper to taste.

Cooking Time: Depending on sausage cooking instructions (usually around 5-7 minutes)

Total Preparation Time: 10 minutes

Serving Size: 1 person

Nutrition Value (per serving):
Calories: Around 300 (depending on sausage and butter)
Protein: Around 20g
Fat: Around 10g
Carbohydrates: Around 30g
Calcium: Small amount from cheese (if added)
Vitamin D: Small amount from fortified bread (if applicable)

Cottage Cheese with Fruit and Nuts

Ingredients:

- 1/2 cup cottage cheese

- 1/2 cup chopped fresh fruit (berries, mango, etc.)

- 2 tablespoons chopped nuts (almonds, walnuts, etc.)

- 1 tablespoon honey (optional)

Preparation Method:

- In a bowl, combine cottage cheese, chopped fruit, and chopped nuts.

- Drizzle with honey (optional) and stir gently to combine.

Total Preparation Time: 5 minutes

Serving Size: 1 person

Nutrition Value (per serving):
Calories: Around 200
Protein: Around 15g

Fat: Around 5g
Carbohydrates: Around 15g (depending on fruit)
Calcium: Around 100mg
Vitamin D: Small amount (if fruit is fortified)
Vitamin C: Good amount from fruits (especially berries)

Chickpea Flour Pancakes with Berries

Ingredients:

- ➢ 1 cup chickpea flour
- ➢ 1 1/2 cups of water, or milk for a more flavorful option
- ➢ 1 tablespoon olive oil
- ➢ 1/2 teaspoon baking powder
- ➢ 1/4 teaspoon salt
- ➢ 1/4 cup fresh berries (blueberries, raspberries, etc.)

Preparation Method:

- In a medium bowl, whisk together chickpea flour, water, olive oil, baking powder, and salt until smooth. Give the batter ten minutes to rest.
- Turn up the heat to medium and gently oil a pan or griddle.
- Pour about 1/4 cup batter per pancake onto the pan.
- Scatter a few berries on top of each pancake batter.
- Cook for 2-3 minutes per side, or until bubbles appear on the surface and the bottom is golden brown. Flip carefully and cook for another 1-2 minutes until cooked through.
- Serve warm with additional berries (optional) and maple syrup or honey (optional).

Cooking Time: 4-5 minutes per pancake (depending on thickness)

Total Preparation Time: 15 minutes

Serving Size: 4-5 pancakes

Nutrition Value (per serving without syrup):
Calories: Around 200
Protein: Around 5g

Fat: Around 5g
Carbohydrates: Around 30g
Calcium: Small amount
Vitamin D: Fortified options may contain some.

Oatmeal with Sliced Almonds and Milk

Ingredients:

- 1/2 cup rolled oats.
- 1 cup milk (dairy or plant-based)
- 1/4 cup water (optional, adjust for desired consistency)
- 1/4 cup sliced almonds.
- 1 tablespoon honey (optional)
- Pinch of cinnamon (optional)

Preparation Method:

- In a saucepan, combine oats, milk, and water (if using).
- Bring to a boil over medium heat, then reduce heat and simmer for 5-7 minutes, or until oats are cooked through and reach desired consistency (add more water if needed).
- Remove from heat and stir in sliced almonds, honey (optional), and cinnamon (optional).

Cooking Time: 5-7 minutes

Total Preparation Time: 10 minutes

Serving Size: 1 person

Nutrition Value (per serving with milk and honey):
Calories: Around 300
Protein: Around 5g
Fat: Around 10g (depending on milk)
Carbohydrates: Around 40g
Calcium: Around 300mg (depending on milk)
Vitamin D: Fortified options may contain some.

Hard-boiled Eggs with Whole-Wheat Toast and Avocado

Ingredients:

- ➢ 2 large eggs
- ➢ 2 slices whole-wheat bread
- ➢ 1/2 ripe avocado, sliced.
- ➢ Salt and pepper to taste

Preparation Method:

- Pour a pan of cold water over the eggs. Put on high heat and bring to a boil.
- Once boiling, remove from heat, cover the pan, and let eggs sit for 10–12 minutes for a medium-cooked yolk. For a harder yolk, cook for an additional 2–3 minutes.
- Meanwhile, toast whole-wheat bread slices to desired doneness.
- Rinse eggs under cold water and peel carefully.
- Spread avocado slices on toasted bread.
- Slice eggs and place them on top of avocado toast. To taste, add salt and pepper for seasoning.

Cooking Time: 10–15 minutes
Total Preparation Time: 15 minutes
Serving Size: 1 person

Nutrition Value (per serving):
Calories: Around 300
Protein: Around 12g
Fat: Around 15g (depending on avocado)
Carbohydrates: Around 20g
Calcium: Around 50mg (per egg)
Vitamin D: Small amount from egg yolk

Lunch recipes.

Chicken Salad Sandwich on Whole-Wheat Bread

Ingredients:

- 2 slices whole-wheat bread
- One cooked and shredded chicken breast, without any bones or flesh
- 1/4 cup mayonnaise (light mayonnaise recommended)
- 1/4 cup chopped celery.
- 1 tablespoon chopped red onion (optional)
- Salt and pepper to taste
- Lettuce leaf (optional)
- Sliced tomato (optional)

Preparation Method:

- Cook boneless, skinless chicken breast according to your preferred method (boiling, baking, grilling, etc.). Let cool and shred the chicken meat.
- In a bowl, combine shredded chicken, mayonnaise, chopped celery, and red onion (if using). To taste, add salt and pepper for seasoning.
- Toast whole-wheat bread slices to desired doneness.
- Spread chicken salad mixture onto one slice of toasted bread.
- Add lettuce and tomato slices (optional) for extra flavor and texture.
- Place the remaining toasted bread slice on top.

Cooking Time: Depends on chicken cooking method (usually 20-30 minutes)

Total Preparation Time: 15 minutes (after chicken is cooked)

Serving Size: 1 sandwich

Nutrition Value (per serving):
Calories: Around 400 (depending on mayonnaise)
Protein: Around 30g
Fat: Around 15g
Carbohydrates: Around 40g

Calcium: Small amount from cheese (if added)
Vitamin D: Small amount from fortified bread (if applicable)

Lentil Soup with Whole-Wheat Bread

Ingredients:

- ➢ 1 cup dry brown lentils
- ➢ 4 cups vegetable broth
- ➢ 1 cup chopped vegetables (carrots, onions, celery, etc.)
- ➢ 1 clove garlic, minced.
- ➢ 1 tablespoon olive oil
- ➢ 1 teaspoon dried thyme
- ➢ 1/2 teaspoon ground cumin
- ➢ Salt and pepper to taste
- ➢ 2 slices whole-wheat bread (optional)

Preparation Method:

- Rinse lentils in a colander.
- In a big pot, warm up the olive oil over medium heat. Add chopped vegetables and garlic. Sauté for 5 minutes, until softened.
- Add lentils, vegetable broth, thyme, and cumin. To taste, add salt and pepper for seasoning.
- Once the lentils are cooked, simmer for 20 to 25 minutes on low heat after bringing to a boil.
- While soup simmers, toast whole-wheat bread slices (optional).

Cooking Time: 25-30 minutes

Total Preparation Time: 35 minutes

Serving Size: 2-3 servings

Nutrition Value (per serving):
Calories: Around 250
Protein: Around 15g

Fat: Around 5g
Carbohydrates: Around 40g
Calcium: Small amount (depending on vegetables)
Vitamin D: Small amount from fortified bread (if applicable)

Tuna Salad with Crackers

Ingredients:

- ➢ 5 oz canned tuna (packed in water)
- ➢ 2 tablespoons mayonnaise (light mayonnaise recommended)
- ➢ 1/4 cup chopped celery.
- ➢ 1 tablespoon chopped red onion (optional)
- ➢ Salt and pepper to taste
- ➢ Whole-wheat crackers

Preparation Method:

- Drain tuna and flake the fish into a bowl.
- Combine tuna with mayonnaise, chopped celery, and red onion (if using). To taste, add salt and pepper for seasoning.
- Serve tuna salad on whole-wheat crackers.

Total Preparation Time: 10 minutes

Serving Size: 1-2 servings

Nutrition Value (per serving, with 6 crackers):
Calories: Around 300
Protein: Around 20g
Fat: Around 10g
Carbohydrates: Around 30g
Calcium: Small amount (depending on crackers)
Vitamin D: Small amount from fortified crackers (if applicable)

Quinoa Bowl with Black Beans and Vegetables

Ingredients:

- 1 cup cooked quinoa
- Rinse and drain one can (15 oz) of black beans.
- 1 cup chopped vegetables (bell peppers, corn, tomatoes, etc.)
- 1/4 cup chopped fresh cilantro.
- 1 tablespoon olive oil
- 1 tablespoon lime juice
- 1/2 teaspoon chili powder (optional)
- Salt and pepper to taste
- Optional toppings: avocado slices, salsa, hot sauce

Preparation Method:

- If not already cooked, prepare quinoa according to package instructions.
- In a bowl, combine cooked quinoa, black beans, chopped vegetables, and fresh cilantro.
- In a separate bowl, whisk together olive oil, lime juice, chili powder (if using), salt, and pepper.
- Drizzle the black bean and quinoa mixture with the dressing. Toss to coat evenly.
- Serve immediately or refrigerate for later.

Cooking Time: Depends on quinoa cooking time (usually around 15 minutes)

Total Preparation Time: 20-25 minutes (including quinoa cooking)

Serving Size: 1 person

Nutrition Value (per serving):
Calories: Around 400 (depending on vegetables and dressing)
Protein: Around 15g
Fat: Around 10g
Carbohydrates: Around 60g
Calcium: Small amount from black beans
Vitamin D: Fortified if using fortified cereal.
Vitamin C: From vegetables (especially tomatoes)

<u>**Salmon Burger on a Whole-Wheat Bun**</u>

Ingredients:

- 1 (6 oz) salmon fillet
- 1/4 cup breadcrumbs (whole-wheat recommended)
- 1 tablespoon chopped onion.
- One tablespoon of freshly chopped dill (or one teaspoon of dried dill)
- 1 egg, beaten.
- 1 tablespoon olive oil
- Whole-wheat hamburger bun
- Lettuce, tomato, red onion slices (optional toppings)
- Mayonnaise, mustard, or yogurt sauce (optional)

Preparation Method:

- In a bowl, combine salmon (flaked with a fork), breadcrumbs, onion, dill, and egg. Season with salt and pepper to taste. Mix well to form a patty.
- Heat olive oil in a pan over medium heat.
- Cook salmon burger for 3-4 minutes per side, or until cooked through and golden brown.
- Toast whole-wheat bun if desired.
- Assemble burger on toasted bun with lettuce, tomato, red onion slices (optional), and your choice of sauce.

Cooking Time: 6-8 minutes

Total Preparation Time: 15-20 minutes

Serving Size: 1 person

Nutrition Value (per serving):
Calories: Around 400 (depending on bun and sauce)
Protein: Around 30g
Fat: Around 20g
Carbohydrates: Around 30g
Calcium: Small amount from bun (if fortified)

| Vitamin D: Small amount from salmon |
| Vitamin C: From vegetables (if used) |

Tofu Veggie Stir-fry with Brown Rice

Ingredients:

- ➢ 1 block firm tofu, drain and press.
- ➢ 1 cup cooked brown rice.
- ➢ 1 cup assorted vegetables (broccoli, carrots, snap peas, etc.)
- ➢ 2 tablespoons soy sauce
- ➢ 1 tablespoon cornstarch
- ➢ 1 tablespoon olive oil
- ➢ 1 clove garlic, minced (optional)
- ➢ 1 teaspoon grated ginger (optional)
- ➢ Salt and pepper to taste

Preparation Method:

- Cut tofu into cubes or small pieces.
- Mix the cornstarch and soy sauce in a small bowl before using.
- On medium-high heat, warm up the olive oil in a big pan or wok.
- Add tofu and cook for a few minutes until slightly browned on all sides.
- Add garlic and ginger (if using) and cook for 30 seconds, stirring constantly.
- Add chopped vegetables and cook for 3-5 minutes, or until tender-crisp.
- Add the soy sauce mixture and whisk until it is well coated. Simmer for a full minute.
- Serve stir-fry over cooked brown rice.

Cooking Time: 10-15 minutes

Total Preparation Time: 20-25 minutes (including brown rice cooking)

Serving Size: 1 person

| Nutrition Value (per serving): |
| Calories: Around 400 (depending on vegetables) |
| Protein: Around 20g |

Fat: Around 10g
Carbohydrates: Around 50g
Calcium: Small amount from tofu
Vitamin D: Fortified if using fortified soy sauce or milk for cooking brown rice.

Greek Yogurt Parfait with Granola and Berries

Ingredients:

- ➢ 1 cup plain Greek yogurt.
- ➢ 1/4 cup granola (preferably low-fat)
- ➢ 1/2 cup fresh berries (blueberries, raspberries, strawberries, etc.)
- ➢ 1 tablespoon honey (optional)

Preparation Method:

- In a bowl or parfait glass, layer half of the Greek yogurt.
- Sprinkle with half of the granola.
- Add half of the berries.
- Repeat layers with remaining yogurt, granola, and berries.
- Drizzle with honey (optional) before serving.

Cooking Time: N/A

Total Preparation Time: 5 minutes

Serving Size: 1 person

Nutrition Value (per serving):
Calories: Around 300 (depending on granola and honey)
Protein: Around 20g
Fat: Around 5g (depending on granola)
Carbohydrates: Around 40g (depending on granola)
Calcium: Around 200mg from yogurt
Vitamin D: Small amount from fortified yogurt (if applicable)
Vitamin C: From fresh berries

Egg Salad Sandwich on Whole-Wheat Pita

Ingredients:

- 2 hard-boiled eggs, chopped.
- 2 tablespoons mayonnaise (light mayonnaise recommended)
- 1 tablespoon chopped celery.
- 1/4 teaspoon dried dill (optional)
- Salt and pepper to taste
- 1 whole-wheat pita bread
- Lettuce and tomato slices (optional)

Preparation Method:

- In a bowl, combine chopped eggs, mayonnaise, celery, dill (if using), salt, and pepper. Mix well.
- Cut the whole-wheat pita bread in half to form a pocket.
- Fill the pita pocket with egg salad mixture.
- Add lettuce and tomato slices (optional) for extra flavor and crunch.

Cooking Time: Depends on egg boiling time (usually around 10-12 minutes)

Total Preparation Time: 15-20 minutes (including egg boiling)

Serving Size: 1 person

Nutrition Value (per serving):
Calories: Around 300 (depending on mayonnaise)
Protein: Around 15g
Fat: Around 15g (depending on mayonnaise)
Carbohydrates: Around 30g
Calcium: Small amount from eggs
Vitamin D: Small amount from eggs
Vitamin C: From vegetables (if used)

Turkey and Cheese Wrap with Vegetables

Ingredients:

- 4 oz sliced deli turkey
- 1 slice cheddar cheese
- 1 whole-wheat tortilla
- 1/4 cup chopped lettuce.
- 1/4 cup chopped tomato.
- 1 tablespoon hummus (optional)
- Salt and pepper to taste

Preparation Method:

- On a platter, spread out the whole-wheat tortilla evenly.
- Spread hummus (optional) on one half of the tortilla.
- Layer lettuce, tomato, and sliced turkey on top of the hummus (or directly on the tortilla if not using hummus).
- Add a slice of cheddar cheese.
- Season with salt and pepper to taste (optional).
- Cover the filling with the bottom of the tortilla folded up. Then, fold in the sides, and roll up tightly to create a wrap.

Total Preparation Time: 5 minutes

Serving Size: 1 person

Nutrition Value (per serving):
Calories: Around 300 (depending on cheese and hummus)
Protein: Around 20g
Fat: Around 10g (depending on cheese and hummus)
Carbohydrates: Around 30g
Calcium: Around 200mg from cheese
Vitamin D: Small amount from cheese (if fortified)
Vitamin C: From vegetables

Chickpea Salad Pita Pockets

Ingredients:

- ➢ 1 (15 oz) can chickpeas, drained and rinsed
- ➢ 1/2 cup chopped vegetables (cucumber, tomato, red onion, etc.)
- ➢ 1/4 cup chopped fresh herbs (parsley, cilantro, mint, etc.)
- ➢ 2 tablespoons olive oil
- ➢ 1 tablespoon lemon juice
- ➢ 1/2 teaspoon ground cumin
- ➢ Salt and pepper to taste
- ➢ 2 whole-wheat pita breads, cut in half.

Preparation Method:

In a bowl, mash the chickpeas with a fork until slightly crumbled. You can leave some whole chickpeas for texture.

Add chopped vegetables, herbs, olive oil, lemon juice, cumin, salt, and pepper. Mix well to combine.

Warm the pita bread halves in a toaster oven or pan for a few minutes until slightly softened.

Instructions:

Spoon the chickpea salad mixture into each pita bread pocket.

Serve immediately.

Cooking Time: N/A (just warming pita bread)

Total Preparation Time: 15-20 minutes

Serving Size: 2 pita pockets

Nutrition Value (per serving):
Calories: Around 300 (depending on vegetables)
Protein: Around 15g
Fat: Around 10g
Carbohydrates: Around 40g
Calcium: Small amount from vegetables
Vitamin D: Fortified if using fortified pita bread

Vitamin C: From vegetables (especially tomatoes)
Iron: From chickpeas

Cheese and Veggie Omelets

Ingredients:

> ➤ 2 eggs
>
> ➤ 1/4 cup shredded cheese (cheddar, mozzarella, etc.)
>
> ➤ 1/2 cup chopped vegetables (spinach, mushrooms, bell peppers, etc.)
>
> ➤ 1 tablespoon butter or olive oil
>
> ➤ Salt and pepper to taste

Preparation Method:

- In a bowl, whisk together eggs with a splash of water or milk. Season with salt and pepper.
- In a pan, preheat the butter or olive oil over medium heat.
- Add chopped vegetables and cook for a few minutes until softened.

Instructions:

- Transfer the egg mixture onto the vegetables in the pan. To evenly distribute the eggs, tilt the pan.
- As the omelette cooks, sprinkle the shredded cheese over one half.
- Once the bottom is set and the top is mostly cooked, use a spatula to fold the omelette in half over the cheese.
- Cook for another minute or two until the cheese is melted and the omelette is cooked through.
- Transfer the omelette to a platter and start serving right away.

Cooking Time: 5-7 minutes

Total Preparation Time: 10-15 minutes

Serving Size: 1 person

Nutrition Value (per serving):
Calories: Around 300 (depending on cheese)
Protein: Around 15g

Fat: Around 15g (depending on butter/oil)
Carbohydrates: Around 5g
Calcium: From cheese and eggs
Vitamin D: Small amount from eggs
Vitamin C: From vegetables (if used)

Dinner recipes

Baked Salmon with Roasted Vegetables

Ingredients:

- ➢ 1 (4-6 oz) salmon fillet
- ➢ 1 tablespoon olive oil
- ➢ 1/2 teaspoon dried herbs (dill, thyme, etc.)
- ➢ Salt and pepper to taste
- ➢ 2 cups assorted vegetables (broccoli, carrots, Brussel sprouts, etc.)
- ➢ 1 tablespoon balsamic vinegar (optional)

Preparation Method:

- Preheat oven to 400°F (200°C).
- Pat salmon dry with paper towels and season with olive oil, dried herbs, salt, and pepper.
- Chop vegetables into bite-sized pieces. Mix them with salt, pepper, and olive oil.
- Arrange veggies in one layer on a baking pan.
- Place salmon fillet on top of the vegetables or beside them on the baking sheet.
- Drizzle vegetables with balsamic vinegar (optional).
- Bake for 15-20 minutes, or until salmon is cooked through and flakes easily with a fork, and vegetables are tender-crisp.

Cooking Time: 15-20 minutes

Total Preparation Time: 20-25 minutes

Serving Size: 1 person

Nutrition Value (per serving):

Calories: Around 400 (depending on vegetables)
Protein: Around 30g
Fat: Around 20g
Carbohydrates: Around 20g
Calcium: Small amount from salmon
Vitamin D: Good amount from salmon

Chicken Stir-fry with Cashews and Brown Rice

Ingredients:

- 1 boneless, skinless chicken breast, sliced.
- 1 cup cooked brown rice.
- 1 cup assorted vegetables (broccoli, carrots, snap peas, etc.)
- 1 tablespoon soy sauce
- 1 tablespoon cornstarch
- 1 tablespoon olive oil
- 1 clove garlic, minced (optional)
- 1/2 cup cashews
- Salt and pepper to taste

Preparation Method:

- Mix the cornstarch and soy sauce in a small bowl before using.
- On medium-high heat, warm up the olive oil in a big pan or wok.
- Add chicken and cook for a few minutes until browned on all sides.
- Add garlic (if using) and cook for 30 seconds, stirring constantly.
- Add chopped vegetables and cook for 3-5 minutes, or until tender-crisp.
- Stir to coat after adding the soy sauce mixture. For one minute, bring to a simmer.
- Stir in cashews and heat through for another minute.
- Serve stir-fry over cooked brown rice.

Cooking Time: 10-15 minutes

Total Preparation Time: 20-25 minutes (including brown rice cooking)

Serving Size: 1 person

Nutrition Value (per serving):
Calories: Around 500 (depending on vegetables)
Protein: Around 30g
Fat: Around 20g
Carbohydrates: Around 50g
Calcium: Small amount from chicken
Vitamin D: Fortified if using fortified soy sauce or milk for cooking brown rice

Lentil Shepherd's Pie

Ingredients:

- 1 cup brown lentils, rinsed.
- 2 cups vegetable broth
- 1 cup chopped vegetables (carrots, onions, celery, etc.)
- 1 tablespoon olive oil
- 1/2 cup cooked peas
- 1/2 cup mashed potatoes (dairy or vegan)
- Salt and pepper to taste
- Optional toppings: chopped fresh herbs (parsley, thyme)

Preparation Method:

- In a medium saucepan, combine lentils and vegetable broth. BOnce the lentils are cooked, simmer for 20 to 25 minutes on low heat after bringing to a boil.
- While lentils are cooking, heat olive oil in a pan over medium heat. Add chopped vegetables and cook for 5-7 minutes, or until softened.
- Drain lentils and mash slightly with a fork (optional).
- Preheat oven to 375°F (190°C).
- In a baking dish, combine cooked lentils, cooked vegetables, and peas. To taste, add salt and pepper for seasoning.
- Top with mashed potatoes, spreading evenly.

- Bake for 20 to 25 minutes, until well cooked and tops begin to turn golden brown.
- Garnish with chopped fresh herbs (optional) before serving.

Cooking Time: 40-45 minutes

Total Preparation Time: 50-55 minutes

Serving Size: 1 person

Nutrition Value (per serving):
Calories: Around 400 (depending on mashed potatoes recipe)
Protein: Around 20g
Fat: Around 10g
Carbohydrates: Around 50g
Calcium: Small amount from lentils
Vitamin D: Fortified if using fortified vegetable broth or milk for mashed potatoes.
Fiber: Good amount from lentils

Turkey Meatloaf with Mashed Sweet Potatoes

- **Ingredients:**
- 1 pound ground turkey (93% lean recommended)
- 1/2 cup chopped onion.
- 1/4 cup chopped celery.
- 1/2 cup grated sweet potato.
- 1/4 cup panko breadcrumbs (whole-wheat recommended)
- 1 large egg, beaten.
- 1 tablespoon Worcestershire sauce
- 1 teaspoon dried thyme
- 1/2 teaspoon salt
- 1/4 teaspoon black pepper
- 1 medium sweet potato, peeled and chopped (for mashed potatoes)
- 1/4 cup milk (dairy or unsweetened plant-based)
- 1 tablespoon butter or olive oil

> Salt and pepper to taste (for mashed potatoes)

Preparation Method:

- Preheat oven to 375°F (190°C). Grease a loaf pan.

- In a large bowl, combine ground turkey, chopped onion, chopped celery, grated sweet potato, panko breadcrumbs, beaten egg, Worcestershire sauce, thyme, salt, and pepper. Mix well to combine.

- Form the mixture into a loaf shape and place it in the prepared loaf pan.

- Bake for 45-50 minutes, or until the internal temperature of the meatloaf reaches 165°F (74°C).

- While the meatloaf is baking, prepare the mashed sweet potatoes. Boil or steam the chopped sweet potato until tender, about 10-15 minutes.

- Drain the cooked sweet potato and mash it with milk and butter or olive oil. To taste, add salt and pepper for seasoning.

Cooking Time: 45-50 minutes for meatloaf, 10-15 minutes for mashed sweet potatoes

Total Preparation Time: 60-70 minutes

Serving Size: 4 (depending on desired portion size)

Nutrition Value (per serving):
Calories: Around 400 (depending on ingredients)
Protein: Around 30g
Fat: Around 20g
Carbohydrates: Around 30g
Vitamin A: High amount from sweet potatoes
Vitamin C: Small amount from vegetables

<u>**Tofu Curry with Vegetables**</u>

Ingredients:

- 1 block firm tofu, drain and press.
- 1 tablespoon olive oil
- 1 onion, chopped.
- 2 cloves garlic, minced.
- 1 teaspoon curry powder
- 1/2 teaspoon turmeric
- 1 (14.5 oz) can diced tomatoes, undrained
- 1 cup vegetable broth
- 1 cup chopped vegetables (broccoli, carrots, bell peppers, etc.)
- 1/4 cup coconut milk (optional)
- 1 tablespoon soy sauce
- 1 tablespoon cornstarch
- Salt and pepper to taste
- Cooked rice (brown or white) for serving.

Preparation Method:

- Cut tofu into cubes or small pieces.
- In a big pot or Dutch oven, warm up the olive oil over medium heat.
- Cook the onion for 3–4 minutes, or until it becomes tender.
- Add garlic, curry powder, and turmeric. Cook for another minute, stirring constantly.
- Stir in diced tomatoes, vegetable broth, and chopped vegetables. Bring to a simmer.
- In a small bowl, whisk together coconut milk (if using), soy sauce, and cornstarch.
- Toss to blend after adding the cornstarch mixture to the saucepan. Spend a few minutes letting the sauce thicken and boil.
- Gently fold in the tofu cubes and heat through for a few more minutes. To taste, add salt and pepper for seasoning.
- Serve tofu curry over cooked rice.

Cooking Time: 20-25 minutes

Total Preparation Time: 30 minutes

Serving Size: 2-3 people

Calories: Around 300 (depending on vegetables and coconut milk)
Protein: Around 20g
Fat: Around 10g
Carbohydrates: Around 30g
Calcium: Small amount from tofu
Vitamin C: From vegetables (especially tomatoes)

White Bean and Kale Soup with Whole-Wheat Bread

Ingredients:

- 1 tablespoon olive oil
- 1 onion, chopped.
- 2 cloves garlic, minced.
- 1 teaspoon dried thyme
- 1/2 teaspoon dried oregano
- 1 (15 oz) can cannellini beans, rinsed and drained
- 1 (15 oz) can white beans, rinsed and drained
- 4 cups vegetable broth
- 4 cups chopped kale.
- Salt and pepper to taste
- 2 slices whole-wheat bread, toasted (optional)
- 1 tablespoon lemon juice (optional)
- Parmesan cheese (optional, for serving)

Preparation Method:

- In a big pot or Dutch oven, warm up the olive oil over medium heat.
- Cook the onion for 3–4 minutes, or until it becomes tender.
- Add garlic, thyme, and oregano. Cook for another minute, stirring constantly.
- Stir in rinsed and drained cannellini beans, white beans, and vegetable broth. After bringing to a boil, lower the heat, and simmer for fifteen minutes.

- Add chopped kale and simmer for another 5-7 minutes, or until kale is wilted and tender.
- Season with salt and pepper to taste.
- Stir in lemon juice (optional) for a brighter flavor.
- Ladle soup into bowls and serve with toasted whole-wheat bread (optional).
- Top with grated Parmesan cheese (optional) for additional flavor.

Cooking Time: 25-30 minutes

Total Preparation Time: 35 minutes

Serving Size: 4-6 people

Nutrition Value (per serving):
Calories: Around 300 (depending on bread and cheese)
Protein: Around 15g
Fat: Around 10g
Carbohydrates: Around 40g
Fiber: Good amount from beans
Calcium: From beans and Parmesan cheese (if used)
Vitamin C: Small amount from vegetables
Vitamin D: Fortified if using fortified vegetable broth.

Baked Cod with Quinoa and Roasted Asparagus

Ingredients:

- 4 cod fillets (4-6 oz each)
- 1 cup quinoa, rinsed.
- 1 1/2 cups vegetable broth
- 1 bunch asparagus, trimmed.
- 1 tablespoon olive oil
- 1/2 lemon, juiced.
- 1/4 teaspoon dried thyme
- Salt and pepper to taste

Preparation Method:

- Preheat oven to 400°F (200°C). Lightly grease a baking dish.
- In a saucepan, combine rinsed quinoa and vegetable broth. Bring to a boil, then reduce heat and simmer for 15 minutes, or until quinoa is cooked and fluffy. Use a fork to fluff, then set aside.
- While the quinoa cooks, prepare the asparagus. Toss asparagus with olive oil, salt, and pepper. Arrange them in a solitary layer on an oven tray.
- Roast the asparagus in the preheated oven for 10-12 minutes, or until tender-crisp.
- Whisk together the lemon juice, olive oil, and thyme in a small basin. Season with salt and pepper.
- Place cod fillets in the prepared baking dish. Brush them with the lemon-herb mixture.
- When the asparagus is done roasting, remove it from the oven and arrange it around the cod fillets in the baking dish.
- Bake the cod for 10-12 minutes, or until the fish flakes easily with a fork and is cooked through.

Cooking Time: 20-24 minutes (10-12 minutes for asparagus, 10-12 minutes for cod)

Total Preparation Time: 35-40 minutes

Serving Size: 4 people

Nutrition Value (per serving):
Calories: Around 400 (depending on oil)
Protein: Around 30g
Fat: Around 15g
Carbohydrates: Around 40g
Vitamin C: Small amount from asparagus
Vitamin D: Small amount from cod

Beef Fajitas with Whole-Wheat Tortillas and Vegetables

Ingredients:

- ➢ 1 pound flank steak thinly sliced.
- ➢ 1 tablespoon olive oil

- ➢ 1 onion thinly sliced.
- ➢ One sliced bell pepper, either red, yellow, or orange
- ➢ 1/2 cup chopped fresh cilantro.
- ➢ 1 lime, juiced.
- ➢ 1 teaspoon chili powder
- ➢ 1/2 teaspoon cumin
- ➢ 1/4 teaspoon smoked paprika (optional)
- ➢ Salt and pepper to taste
- ➢ 4 whole-wheat tortillas, warmed.
- ➢ Add-ons: sour cream, salsa, guacamole, and shredded cheese

Preparation Method:

- In a large bowl, combine sliced flank steak with olive oil, chili powder, cumin, smoked paprika (if using), salt, and pepper. Toss to coat the meat evenly.
- A big skillet or grill pan should be heated to medium-high heat. Add the marinated steak and cook for 3-4 minutes per side, or until desired doneness. Steak should be taken out of the pan and placed aside.
- In the same pan, add the sliced onion and bell pepper. Cook for 5-7 minutes, or until softened and slightly browned.
- Stir in chopped cilantro and lime juice.
- Slice the cooked steak into thin strips.
- Warm whole-wheat tortillas according to package instructions (microwave, stovetop, etc.)

Cooking Time: 8-10 minutes (depending on steak thickness and desired doneness)

Total Preparation Time: 20-25 minutes

Serving Size: 4 people

Nutrition Value (per serving):
Calories: Around 400 (depending on toppings)
Protein: Around 30g
Fat: Around 20g
Carbohydrates: Around 30g

Vitamin C: From vegetables and lime juice

Chickpea Fritters with Yogurt Dill Sauce

Ingredients:

- 1 cup cooked and overnight-soaked dry chickpeas.
- 1/4 cup chopped onion.
- 1/4 cup chopped fresh parsley.
- 1 tablespoon olive oil
- 1/2 teaspoon ground cumin
- 1/4 teaspoon chili powder (optional)
- 1/4 cup chickpea flour (gram flour)
- Salt and pepper to taste

For the Yogurt Dill Sauce:

- 1 cup plain Greek yogurt.
- 1/4 cup chopped fresh dill.
- 1 tablespoon lemon juice
- 1/4 teaspoon garlic powder (optional)
- Salt and pepper to taste

Preparation Method:

- Drain and rinse the cooked chickpeas.
- In a food processor, combine chickpeas, onion, parsley, olive oil, cumin, chili powder (if using), and chickpea flour. Pulse until a slightly coarse mixture forms. To taste, add salt and pepper for seasoning.
- In a pan, heat a thin layer of oil over medium heat.
- Scoop the chickpea mixture by tablespoons and form into small patties.
- Fry the fritters for 2-3 minutes per side, or until golden brown and crispy.
- While the fritters are cooking, prepare the yogurt dill sauce. In a bowl, whisk together Greek yogurt, chopped dill, lemon juice, garlic powder (if using), salt, and pepper.

Cooking Time: 5-7 minutes for frying the fritters

Total Preparation Time: 30-35 minutes (including soaking chickpeas)

Serving Size: 4-6 fritters

Nutrition Value (per serving, without sauce):
Calories: Around 200
Protein: Around 10g
Fat: Around 5g
Carbohydrates: Around 30g
Fiber: Good amount from chickpeas
Yogurt Dill Sauce Nutrition (per serving):
Calories: Around 50
Protein: Around 5g
Fat: Around 0g
Carbohydrates: Around 5g

Brown rice and black beans accompanied by cheese enchiladas.

Ingredients:

- 1 cup cooked brown rice.
- 1 (15 oz) can black beans, rinsed and drained
- One cup of shredded cheese, such as Monterey Jack or cheddar
- 1/2 cup enchilada sauce
- 4 corn tortillas
- 1/4 cup chopped onion (optional)
- 1 clove garlic, minced (optional)
- 1/4 cup chopped fresh cilantro (optional)
- Canola oil for cooking

Preparation Method:

- Preheat oven to 375°F (190°C). Lightly grease a baking dish.
- In a bowl, combine cooked brown rice, black beans, and 1/2 cup of the shredded cheese. Season with salt and pepper to taste (optional).

- If using, heat a little oil in a pan over medium heat. Sauté chopped onion and garlic for a few minutes until softened. Add them to the rice and black bean mixture.

- Divide the rice and bean mixture evenly amongst the 4 tortillas. Roll them up tightly.

- After the baking dish is ready, put the rolled enchiladas seam-side down.

- Pour the enchilada sauce over the enchiladas, coating them evenly.

- Sprinkle the remaining shredded cheese on top.

- Bake for 20-25 minutes, or until heated through and cheese is melted and bubbly.

- Garnish with chopped fresh cilantro (optional) before serving.

Cooking Time: 20-25 minutes

Total Preparation Time: 30-35 minutes (including cooking brown rice)

Serving Size: 4 enchiladas

Nutrition Value (per serving):
Calories: Around 400 (depending on cheese and enchilada sauce)
Protein: Around 20g
Fat: Around 15g
Carbohydrates: Around 40g
Calcium: From cheese
Fiber: From black beans and brown rice

Snacks recipes

Fruit and Yogurt Parfait

Ingredients:

- 1 cup plain yogurt (Greek yogurt recommended for extra protein)
- 1/2 cup chopped fresh fruit (berries, mango, etc.)
- 1/4 cup granola (optional)
- 1 tablespoon honey (optional)

Preparation Method:

- In a bowl or parfait glass, layer yogurt and chopped fruit.

- Add granola (optional) for a crunchy texture.
- Drizzle with honey (optional) for extra sweetness.

Total Preparation Time: 5 minutes

Serving Size: 1 person

Nutrition Value (per serving, using plain yogurt and berries):
Calories: Around 200
Protein: Around 10g (more with Greek yogurt)
Fat: Around 5g
Carbohydrates: Around 30g
Calcium: Around 300mg (more with Greek yogurt)
Vitamin C: Good amount from berries

Trail mix contains almonds, raisins, and sunflower seeds.

Ingredients:

- 1/2 cup raw almonds
- 1/2 cup raisins
- 1/4 cup sunflower seeds
- You can also add other ingredients like dried fruit (cranberries, chopped dates, etc.), nuts (cashews, walnuts, pistachios), or dark chocolate chips (optional).

Preparation Method:

- In a bowl, combine almonds, raisins, and sunflower seeds.
- If using additional ingredients, add them to the mix and stir well.

Total Preparation Time: 5 minutes

Serving Size: 1 person (can be adjusted depending on desired portion size)

Nutrition Value (per serving):
Calories: Around 200 (depending on ingredients)
Protein: Around 5g
Fat: Around 10g

Carbohydrates: Around 25g
Fiber: Good amount from nuts and raisins
Iron: From almonds and sunflower seeds

Hard-boiled Egg with Sliced Apple

Ingredients:

- ➢ 1 large egg
- ➢ 1 apple, sliced.

Preparation Method:

- Place the egg in a saucepan and fill with cold water.
- Bring the water to a boil, then remove from heat and cover the pot for 10-12 minutes for a medium-hard-boiled egg. (Adjust cooking time for desired doneness: 7-8 minutes for soft-boiled, 13-15 minutes for hard-boiled)
- While the egg is cooking, slice the apple.
- Remove the egg from the hot water and place it in a bowl of cold water for at least 5 minutes to stop the cooking process.
- Peel the egg and enjoy it with sliced apple.

Cooking Time: 10-15 minutes (depending on desired doneness)

Total Preparation Time: 15 minutes

Serving Size: 1 person

Nutrition Value (per serving):
Calories: Around 150
Protein: Around 6g (from egg)
Fat: Around 5g (from egg)
Carbohydrates: Around 25g (from apple)
Vitamin C: From apple
Choline: From egg (important for brain health)

Cottage Cheese with Pineapple Chunks

Ingredients:

- 1/2 cup cottage cheese
- 1/2 cup chopped fresh pineapple.
- 1 tablespoon chopped nuts (almonds, walnuts, etc.) (optional)
- 1 tablespoon honey (optional)

Preparation Method:

- In a bowl, combine cottage cheese and chopped pineapple.
- Add chopped nuts (optional) for extra protein and texture.
- Drizzle with honey (optional) for sweetness.

Total Preparation Time: 5 minutes

Serving Size: 1 person

Nutrition Value (per serving):
Calories: Around 200
Protein: Around 15g
Fat: Around 5g
Carbohydrates: Around 20g
Vitamin C: From pineapple
Calcium: Around 100mg

Edamame Pods

Ingredients:

- 1 cup frozen edamame pods (shelled or in pods)
- Water
- Salt (optional)

Preparation Method:

- If using frozen shelled edamame:
- Heat a saucepan of water until it boils.
- Add edamame pods and cook for 3-5 minutes, or until tender-crisp.
- Drain the water.

- If using frozen edamame pods in pods:

- Thaw the pods in a colander under running cold water for a few minutes.

- Heat up some salted water in a pot.

- Add edamame pods and cook for 5-7 minutes, or until pods turn bright green and the beans are tender-crisp.

- Drain the water and sprinkle the pods with a little salt (optional).

- Pinch or twist the pods open to remove the edamame beans.

Cooking Time: 3-7 minutes

Total Preparation Time: 5-10 minutes

Serving Size: 1 person (as a snack)

Nutrition Value (per serving):
Calories: Around 120
Protein: Around 15g
Fat: Around 5g
Carbohydrates: Around 10g
Fiber: Good amount
Vitamin C: Small amount

Bean and Veggie Salad

Ingredients:

- 1 cup cooked beans (chickpeas, kidney beans, black beans, etc.)
- 1 cup chopped vegetables (chopped tomatoes, bell peppers, cucumbers, etc.)
- 1/4 cup chopped red onion (optional)
- 1 tablespoon olive oil
- 1 tablespoon vinegar (red wine vinegar, balsamic vinegar, etc.)
- 1/2 teaspoon dried herbs (Italian seasoning, oregano, etc.) (optional)
- Salt and pepper to taste

Preparation Method:

- In a bowl, combine cooked beans and chopped vegetables.

- Add chopped red onion (optional).
- In a separate bowl, whisk together olive oil, vinegar, dried herbs (if using), salt, and pepper.
- Over the bean and vegetable combination, drizzle the dressing.
- Toss to coat evenly.

Cooking Time: Depends on bean cooking time (usually 15-20 minutes for dried beans)

Total Preparation Time: 15-20 minutes (not including bean cooking time)

Serving Size: 1 person (as a side dish)

Nutrition Value (per serving):
Calories: Around 200 (depending on ingredients)
Protein: Around 10g
Fat: Around 5g
Carbohydrates: Around 30g
Fiber: Good amount from beans
Vitamin C: From vegetables (especially tomatoes)

Orange with Sliced Almonds

Ingredients:

- 1 orange
- 1/4 cup sliced almonds.

Preparation Method:

- Wash and dry the orange.
- Peel the orange, removing the white pith as much as possible.
- Segment the orange by cutting between the membranes to separate the orange flesh.
- Alternatively, you can slice the orange into rounds.

Total Preparation Time: 5 minutes

Serving Size: 1 person (as a snack)

Nutrition Value (per serving):

Calories: Around 70
Protein: Around 1g
Fat: Around 0g
Carbohydrates: Around 15g
Vitamin C: High amount from orange
Healthy Fats: From almonds

Yogurt with Berries and Pumpkin Seeds

Ingredients:

- ➢ 1 cup plain yogurt (Greek yogurt recommended for extra protein)
- ➢ 1/2 cup fresh berries (blueberries, raspberries, strawberries, etc.)
- ➢ 2 tablespoons pumpkin seeds

Preparation Method:

- In a bowl, combine plain yogurt and fresh berries.
- Sprinkle pumpkin seeds on top.

Total Preparation Time: 2 minutes

Serving Size: 1 person

Nutrition Value (per serving, using plain yogurt):
Calories: Around 200
Protein: Around 10g (more with Greek yogurt)
Fat: Around 5g
Carbohydrates: Around 30g
Calcium: Around 300mg (more with Greek yogurt)
Vitamin C: Good amount from berries

Whole-Wheat Crackers with Cheese

Ingredients:

- ➢ 4 whole-wheat crackers
- ➢ 2 slices of cheese (cheddar, swiss, mozzarella, etc.)

Preparation Method:

- Place whole-wheat crackers on a plate.
- Top each cracker with a slice of cheese.

Total Preparation Time: 1 minute

Serving Size: 1 person

Nutrition Value (per serving, using cheddar cheese):
Calories: Around 200 (depending on cheese)
Protein: Around 8g
Fat: Around 10g
Carbohydrates: Around 20g
Calcium: Around 200mg (depending on cheese)
Vitamin D: Small amount from cheese (if fortified)

Milk and Fortified Cereal

Ingredients:

- ➢ 1 cup milk (dairy or fortified plant-based)
- ➢ 1 serving of fortified cereal (flakes, granola, etc.)

Preparation Method:

- Pour milk into a bowl.
- Add a serving of fortified cereal.

Total Preparation Time: 1 minute

Serving Size: 1 person

Nutrition Value (per serving, using whole-wheat flakes cereal and dairy milk):
Calories: Around 200 (depending on cereal)

Protein: Around 8g
Fat: Around 5g
Carbohydrates: Around 30g
Calcium: Around 300mg (from milk)
Vitamin D: Fortified in milk and cereal
Fiber: Good amount from whole-wheat cereal (if used)

14 days bone strength meal plan

Day 1:

Breakfast: Scrambled Eggs with Kale and Cheese
Lunch: Chicken Salad Sandwich on Whole-Wheat Bread
Dinner: Baked Salmon with Roasted Vegetables
Snack: Trail Mix with Almonds, Raisins, and Sunflower Seeds

Day 2

Breakfast: High-Protein Yogurt Bowl
Lunch: Lentil Soup with Whole-Wheat Bread
Dinner: Chicken Stir-fry with Cashews and Brown Rice
Snack: Cottage Cheese with Pineapple Chunks

Day 3:

Breakfast: Tofu Scramble with Bell Peppers
Lunch: Tuna Salad with Crackers
Dinner: Lentil Shepherd's Pie

Snack: Fruit and Yogurt Parfait

Day 4:

Breakfast: Fortified Cereal with Milk and Fruit
Lunch: Quinoa Bowl with Black Beans and Vegetables
Dinner: Turkey Meatloaf with Mashed Sweet Potatoes
Snack: Bean and Veggie Salad

Day 5:

Breakfast: Salmon and Veggie Frittata
Lunch: Greek Yogurt Parfait with Granola and Berries
Dinner: Tofu Curry with Vegetables
Snack: Hard-boiled Egg with Sliced Apple

Day 6:

Breakfast: Nut Butter and Banana Smoothie
Lunch: Egg Salad Sandwich on Whole-Wheat Pita
Dinner: White Bean and Kale Soup with Whole-Wheat Bread
Snack: Yogurt with Berries and Pumpkin Seeds

Day 7:

Breakfast: Turkey Sausage and Whole-Wheat Toast
Lunch: Turkey and Cheese Wrap with Vegetables
Dinner: Baked Cod with Quinoa and Roasted Asparagus
Snack: Whole-Wheat Crackers with Cheese

Day 8 (Relaxation Day - leftovers or simple meals):

Choose any breakfast, lunch, or dinner recipe you enjoyed earlier in the week, or opt for something quick and easy. Pick one snack you like from the options provided.

Day 9:

Breakfast: Chickpea Flour Pancakes with Berries

Lunch: Chickpea Salad Pita Pockets

Dinner: Beef Fajitas with Whole-Wheat Tortillas and Vegetables

Snack: Edamame Pods

Day 10:

Breakfast: Oatmeal with Sliced Almonds and Milk

Lunch: Cheese and Veggie Omelette

Dinner: Chickpea Fritters with Yogurt Dill Sauce

Snack: Orange with Sliced Almonds

Day 11:

Breakfast: Hard-boiled Eggs with Whole-Wheat Toast and Avocado

Lunch: Chicken Salad Sandwich on Whole-Wheat Bread (repeat, for protein balance)

Dinner: Tofu Curry with Vegetables (repeat, for a different protein source)

Snack: Milk and Fortified Cereal

Day 12:

Breakfast: Fortified Cereal with Milk and Fruit (repeat, for ease)

Lunch: Lentil Soup with Whole-Wheat Bread (repeat, as it's a vegetarian option)

Dinner: Baked Salmon with Roasted Vegetables (repeat, as it's a good source of omega-3 fatty acids)
Snack: Cottage Cheese with Fruit and Nuts

Breakfast: Nut Butter and Banana Smoothie (repeat, for a quick and filling option)
Lunch: Tuna Salad with Crackers (repeat, for ease)
Dinner: Chicken Stir-fry with Cashews and Brown Rice (repeat, for a quick and easy option)
Snack: Fruit and Yogurt Parfait

Breakfast: Scrambled Eggs with Kale and Cheese (repeat, as it's a protein-rich option)
Lunch: Leftovers or choose any recipe you enjoyed earlier in the week
Dinner: Choose any dinner recipe you enjoyed earlier in the week
Snack: Trail Mix with Almonds, Raisins, and Sunflower Seeds

Tips for Incorporating Calcium-Rich Foods into Pregnancy Diet

Strengthening Bones for Two: Calcium in Pregnancy

Calcium is crucial for building strong bones in both you and your developing baby. During pregnancy, your body uses calcium to support fetal skeletal development. *Here's how to incorporate calcium-rich foods into your diet:*

- **Dairy Delights:** opt for low-fat or fat-free milk, yogurt, and cheese. Two cups of milk provide nearly 700mg of calcium, fulfilling most of your daily needs. Yogurt offers protein alongside calcium, making it a power-packed snack. Choose cheese with moderation, opting for lower-sodium varieties.

- **Leafy Green Powerhouse:** Don't underestimate the power of dark, leafy greens like kale, collard greens, and spinach. While they contain less calcium per serving compared to dairy, they are packed with vitamins and minerals that aid calcium absorption.

- **Fish with a Bonus:** Fatty fish like sardines and salmon are excellent sources of calcium and vitamin D, another essential nutrient for bone health. Canned sardines, eaten with soft bones, offer a surprising calcium boost.

- **Fortified Fun:** Many breakfast cereals and plant-based milks are fortified with calcium. Look for options with at least 30% of your Daily Value (DV) per serving.

Remember, a balanced diet is key. By incorporating these calcium-rich options, you're ensuring a healthy foundation for both you and your growing baby.

Prenatal Vitamins and Bone Health:

Building a Strong Foundation

Try to understand the importance of bone health during pregnancy. Not only are you nourishing yourself, but you're also building a strong skeletal system for your developing baby. Vitamins for pregnancy are essential to this process.

Prenatal Powerhouse:

Prenatal vitamins are a targeted supplement containing essential vitamins and minerals,

including:

Calcium is the building block of bones. It's crucial for fetal bone development and maintaining your own bone density.

Vitamin D aids in calcium absorption from the gut. Deficiency can hinder your baby's bone growth and increase your risk of pregnancy-related complications.

Folic acid: Lowers the baby's chance of neural tube abnormalities.

Iron supports fetal development and red blood cell production.

Other vitamins and minerals play vital roles in overall health.

Calcium and Vitamin D Supplements: Weighing the Benefits:

Calcium:

Benefits: Ensures adequate calcium intake for fetal bone development and helps maintain your bone density, especially if dietary intake is insufficient.

Considerations: High doses can interfere with iron absorption. Discuss the optimal dosage with your doctor based on your individual needs and dietary habits.

Vitamin D:

Benefits: Essential for calcium absorption and promoting bone mineralization in your baby. It also supports a healthy immune system in both of you.

Considerations: Vitamin D deficiency is common, especially in pregnant women. Regular blood tests may be needed to monitor vitamin D levels and determine if supplementation is necessary.

Ready to talk about keeping those bones strong and healthy. Now, before you doze off like in a lecture hall, imagine your skeleton as your personal superhero suit—you got to keep it sturdy, right? So, let's dive into some key practices that'll have your bones thanking you later.

First up: Smoking Cessation—Kicking the Butt for Bone's Sake!

Picture this: you light up a cigarette, and with that puff, tiny ninjas wielding smoke bombs invade your bones! They weaken the structure, making them more susceptible to fractures. Scary, huh? Well, that's essentially what happens when you smoke. The nicotine disrupts the natural bone-building process, making them thinner and more brittle. So, ditch the smokes! Think of it as an upgrade to your internal superhero suit – a smoke-free, bone-strengthening shield!

Alcohol Limitation: Friend or Foe to Bones?

Now, let's talk about alcohol. Imagine your bones are having a pool party. A little bit of fun is okay (think a light beer) – it might even help with stress reduction, which we'll get to in a bit. But too much partying (think of several cocktails) is like inviting a bunch of rowdy bone-dissolving gremlins to the bash. They disrupt calcium absorption and mess with hormone production, both crucial for bone health. So, keep the alcohol intake moderate – your bones will thank you for it, and you'll avoid a nasty hangover as a bonus!

Weight Management: Not Just About the Beach Bod

Let's face it, maintaining a healthy weight is like having a skilled engineer overseeing your bone construction site. When you're overweight or obese, it puts extra stress on your bones, especially in weight-bearing areas like the hips and knees. Think of it as overloading a bridge – it can eventually start to crack. But the good news is, even modest weight loss can significantly improve bone health! So, ditch the fad diets and focus on a balanced lifestyle with healthy eating and exercise – your bones will be your strongest supporters (pun intended).

Stress Reduction Techniques: Keeping Your Bones Chill

Stress can act like a sneaky thief, stealing calcium from your bones. Imagine you're stressed, and tiny, frantic squirrels are hoarding all the calcium in your body! Not ideal, right? So, finding healthy ways to manage stress is key for bone health. Try some deep breathing exercises, meditation, yoga – anything that helps you unwind and keeps those squirrels at bay. Bonus points if you find something that makes you laugh – laughter truly is the best medicine, and it helps reduce stress hormones too!

Remember, folks, keeping your bones strong is an investment in your future health. By following these tips, you'll be well on your way to a healthy, active life – with a superhero skeleton to boot!

Addressing Bone Health Concerns After Childbirth

Imagine your bones as a bank account. During pregnancy, your little tenant-in-training starts withdrawing calcium to build their own strong skeleton. This can leave your account a bit depleted. Now, the good news is your body is amazing, and it starts naturally redepositing calcium after birth. But sometimes, that process needs a little help, especially if you have a risk factor like low pre-pregnancy calcium intake, a history of fractures, or certain medical conditions.

Strategies for Maintaining Bone Density

So, how do we keep those bones feeling like a fortress and not a cracker waiting to crumble?

Here are some key strategies:

<u>Calcium is Your BFF:</u> We're talking dairy delights like low-fat yogurt (think creamy parfaits!), cheese (go for the string cheese for a fun, low-mess snack!), and of course, milk (ditch the sugary drinks and guzzle some calcium instead!). Don't forget those leafy greens – kale chips anyone? They may not be birthday cake, but they're a nutritional powerhouse for your bones.

<u>Vitamin D is the Sunshine Partner:</u> Vitamin D helps your body absorb calcium, so think sunshine (soak up those safe rays!) or grab some vitamin D-fortified foods like salmon (think fancy dinner with a side of bone health!) or fortified cereals.

<u>Weight-Bearing Exercise is Your Superhero Training:</u> Remember all those superhero landings you practiced while chasing your little one? Turns out, weight-bearing exercises like walking, hiking, or even dancing with your baby are fantastic for bone health. Think of it as building those superhero bones, one step (or shimmy) at a time!

Postpartum Nutrition and Exercise Recommendations

Now, listen up, mama! Here's the deal: after childbirth, your body is recovering, and it needs all the fuel it can get. Don't go on a crash diet – your bones (and your sanity!) will thank you. Aim for a balanced diet with plenty of fruits, vegetables, whole grains, and lean protein. And remember, gentle exercise is your friend. Start slow and gradually increase the intensity as your body allows.

Remember: Don't be afraid to talk to your doctor about any specific concerns you have about your bone health. They can help you create a personalized plan to keep those bones strong and ready for all the adventures you and your little one will have together.

The Cornerstone of a Healthy Pregnancy: Prenatal Care and Regular Check-Ups

It's the foundation for a healthy pregnancy journey for both you and your baby. Regular check-ups throughout your pregnancy allow you to monitor your health, identify potential risks early on, and ensure the optimal development of your little one.

Think of prenatal care as a roadmap. It provides a structured approach to your pregnancy, allowing to:

Confirm pregnancy and track its development: We'll use scans and tests to confirm the pregnancy, monitor fetal growth, and detect any potential abnormalities early on.

Screen for health risks: We can screen for conditions like gestational diabetes, preeclampsia, and chromosomal abnormalities, allowing for early intervention if necessary.

Address your health concerns: Prenatal visits are a safe space to discuss any questions, anxieties, or physical issues you may be experiencing.

Educate you on pregnancy: We'll provide information on nutrition, exercise, and lifestyle modifications to support a healthy pregnancy.

Prepare you for childbirth: Prenatal visits also include discussions about birthing options, pain management techniques, and postpartum care.

Regular check-ups allow for personalized care that adapts to your unique needs. By building a strong relationship with your healthcare team, you can feel confident and empowered throughout your pregnancy.

Obstetricians, Dietitians, and Bone Health Specialists

A successful pregnancy journey often involves a collaborative effort between several healthcare professionals. Here's a breakdown of some key members of your pregnancy team:

Obstetrician (OB-GYN): Your OB-GYN is your primary care provider during pregnancy. They'll conduct prenatal check-ups, order necessary tests, and manage your overall health throughout the journey.

Registered Dietitian (RD): A registered dietitian can create a personalized nutrition plan to ensure you and your baby receive the essential nutrients for optimal development. They can address any dietary restrictions you may have and provide guidance on healthy pregnancy weight gain.

 In some cases, your doctor may recommend consulting a bone health specialist. This could be particularly relevant if you have a history of osteoporosis or other bone health concerns. They can advise on strategies to maximize calcium absorption and maintain your skeletal health during pregnancy.

Common Concerns and Myths

Dispelling Myths Surrounding Osteoporosis and Pregnancy

It's a common misconception that pregnancy weakens your bones and leads to osteoporosis. Let's dispel the following myths:

Myth 1: Pregnancy "steals" calcium from your bones, weakening them.

This isn't entirely true. While your developing baby does need calcium for bone growth, your body prioritizes fetal health. It increases your calcium absorption from food and releases hormones to maintain bone density.

Myth 2: Having children increases your risk of osteoporosis later in life.

The number of pregnancies you have doesn't directly increase your osteoporosis risk. However, other factors like genetics, low calcium intake throughout life, and certain medical conditions can play a role.

Myth 3: Breastfeeding causes osteoporosis.

There's no evidence to support this. While some calcium is transferred to your baby through breast milk, your body continues to adjust and maintain bone health.

Empowering Bone Health During Pregnancy

Pregnancy marks a time of incredible transformation. As your body nurtures a new life, your bones play a vital role in providing the building blocks for your baby's skeletal development. However, for women with pre-existing bone conditions like osteoporosis, this period can raise concerns about bone health.

Throughout this text, we've explored the unique challenges faced by expecting mothers with pre-existing bone conditions. We've discussed the increased calcium demands, hormonal shifts, and additional weight strain placed on the bones during pregnancy. We've also explored into the complexities of managing osteoporosis when other health conditions are present, highlighting the importance of medication adjustments, monitoring underlying conditions, and managing potential joint pain.

Summary of Key Takeaways:

Women with pre-existing bone conditions require careful planning and collaboration with their healthcare team before and during pregnancy.

Pre-pregnancy consultations allow for assessment of individual risk factors and development of personalized bone health strategies.

Calcium and vitamin D supplementation, proper weight management, weight-bearing exercises, and a balanced diet rich in calcium sources are crucial for maintaining bone health during pregnancy.

Open communication with your doctor regarding concerns, potential complications, and adjustments to medications is essential when managing osteoporosis alongside other health conditions.

Empowerment and Advocacy for Bone Health:

Knowledge is power. By understanding how your body changes during pregnancy and how potential bone conditions might be affected, you can become an active participant in your own healthcare journey. There are many resources available to women facing similar challenges. Support groups, online communities, and bone health organizations can provide valuable information and connections with others who understand your experiences.

You Are Not Alone

Building a healthy foundation for your growing baby is a noble and empowering endeavor. Remember that you are not alone on this path. With proactive planning, open communication with your healthcare team, and a commitment to bone health, you can navigate pregnancy with confidence. Embrace these steps towards empowered motherhood, knowing that every effort you make contributes to a strong and healthy future for both you and your child.

The journey of pregnancy requires resilience and a commitment to your own well-being. By prioritizing bone health and advocating for your needs, you can pave the way for a healthy and joyful pregnancy experience. Remember, a strong foundation starts with you, and the steps you take today will benefit generations to come.

WELCOME TO THE BONUS SECTION

Two amazing bonuses await you as you explore this section.

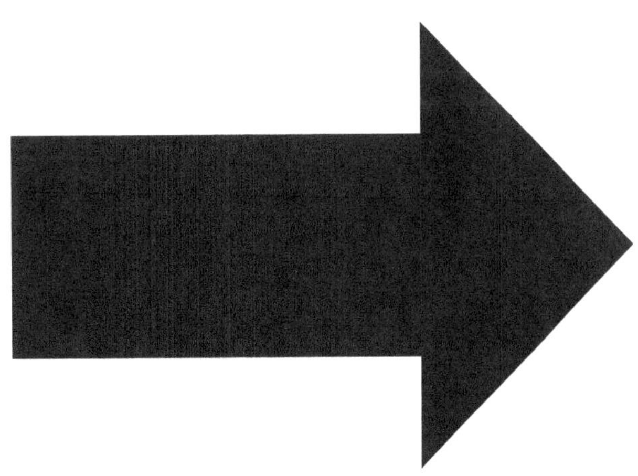

 # WEEKLY MEAL PLANNER 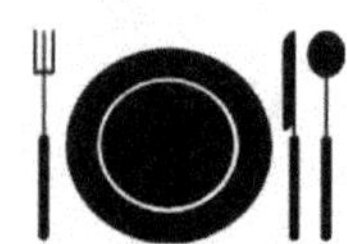

WEEK ______________________

	BREAKFAST	LUNCH	DINNER	SNACKS
MON				
TUE				
WED				
THU				
FRI				
SAT				
SUN				

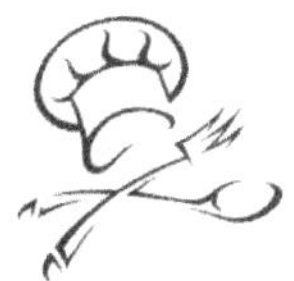 # WEEKLY MEAL PLANNER 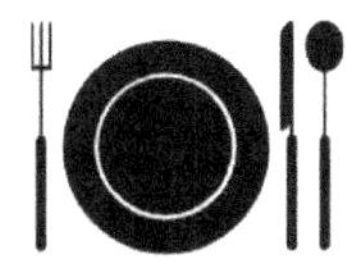

WEEK

	BREAKFAST	LUNCH	DINNER	SNACKS
MON				
TUE				
WED				
THU				
FRI				
SAT				
SUN				

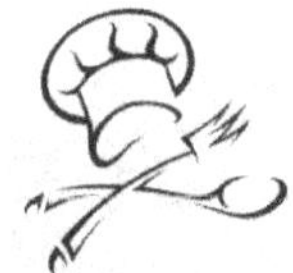# WEEKLY MEAL PLANNER 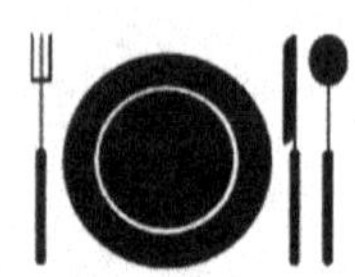

WEEK ___________

	BREAKFAST	LUNCH	DINNER	SNACKS
MON				
TUE				
WED				
THU				
FRI				
SAT				
SUN				

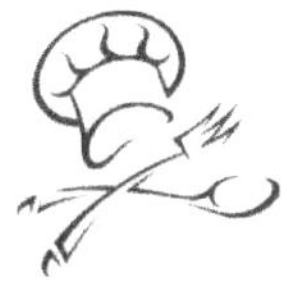 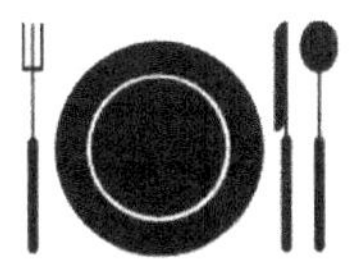

WEEKLY MEAL PLANNER

WEEK

	BREAKFAST	LUNCH	DINNER	SNACKS
MON				
TUE				
WED				
THU				
FRI				
SAT				
SUN				

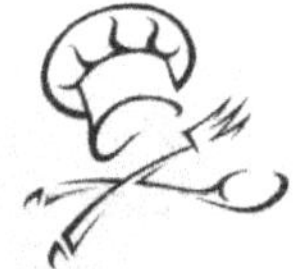 # WEEKLY MEAL PLANNER 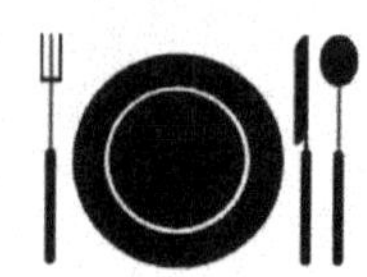

WEEK ___________________________

	BREAKFAST	LUNCH	DINNER	SNACKS
MON				
TUE				
WED				
THU				
FRI				
SAT				
SUN				

 # WEEKLY MEAL PLANNER 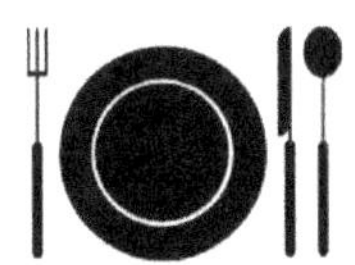

WEEK

	BREAKFAST	LUNCH	DINNER	SNACKS
MON				
TUE				
WED				
THU				
FRI				
SAT				
SUN				

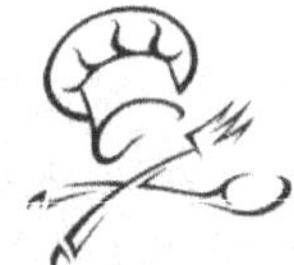# WEEKLY MEAL PLANNER 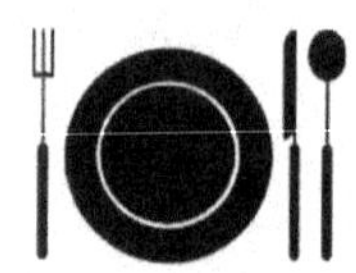

WEEK

	BREAKFAST	LUNCH	DINNER	SNACKS
MON				
TUE				
WED				
THU				
FRI				
SAT				
SUN				

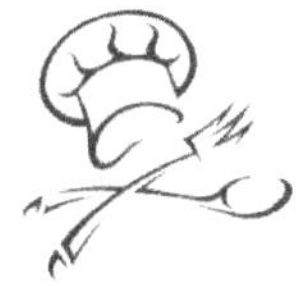 # WEEKLY MEAL PLANNER 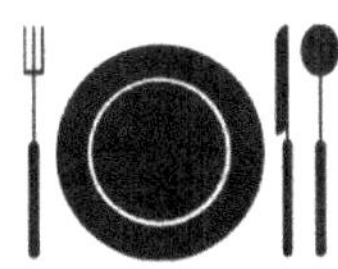

WEEK

	BREAKFAST	LUNCH	DINNER	SNACKS
MON				
TUE				
WED				
THU				
FRI				
SAT				
SUN				

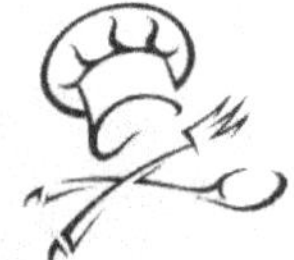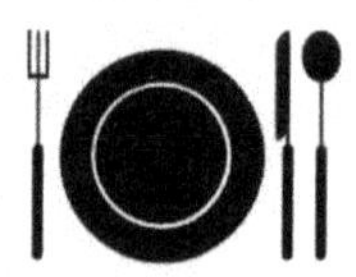

WEEKLY MEAL PLANNER

WEEK

	BREAKFAST	LUNCH	DINNER	SNACKS
MON				
TUE				
WED				
THU				
FRI				
SAT				
SUN				

 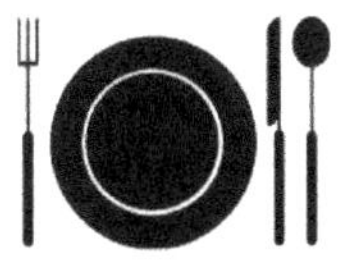

WEEKLY MEAL PLANNER

WEEK

	BREAKFAST	LUNCH	DINNER	SNACKS
MON				
TUE				
WED				
THU				
FRI				
SAT				
SUN				

Efficient Work Log for Expectant Moms

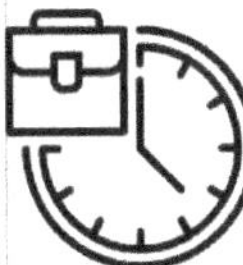 

WORK LOG

MONTH:

DATE	WORK ACTIVITY	START TIME	END TIME		TOTAL HOURS
		:	:		
		:	:		
		:	:		
		:	:		
		:	:		
		:	:		
		:	:		
		:	:		
		:	:		
		:	:		
		:	:		
		:	:		
		:	:		
		:	:		
		:	:		
		:	:		

NOTE:

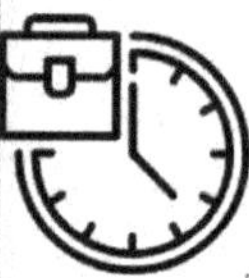

WORK LOG

MONTH:

DATE	WORK ACTIVITY	START TIME	END TIME		TOTAL HOURS
		:	:		
		:	:		
		:	:		
		:	:		
		:	:		
		:	:		
		:	:		
		:	:		
		:	:		
		:	:		
		:	:		
		:	:		
		:	:		
		:	:		
		:	:		
		:	:		

NOTE:

WORK LOG

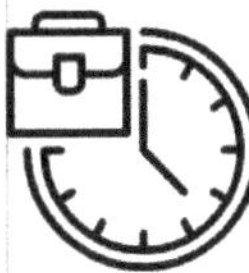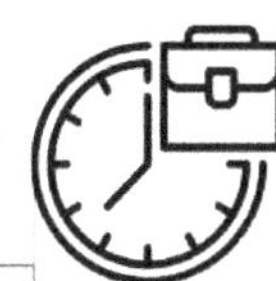

MONTH:

DATE	WORK ACTIVITY	START TIME	END TIME		TOTAL HOURS
		:	:		
		:	:		
		:	:		
		:	:		
		:	:		
		:	:		
		:	:		
		:	:		
		:	:		
		:	:		
		:	:		
		:	:		
		:	:		
		:	:		
		:	:		
		:	:		

NOTE:

WORK LOG

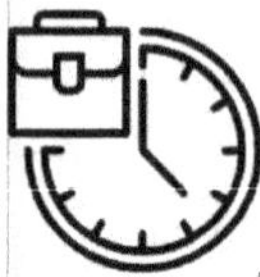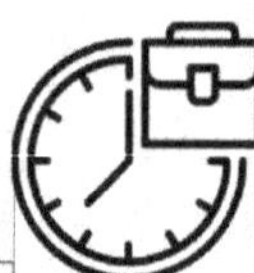

MONTH:

DATE	WORK ACTIVITY	START TIME	END TIME		TOTAL HOURS
		:	:		
		:	:		
		:	:		
		:	:		
		:	:		
		:	:		
		:	:		
		:	:		
		:	:		
		:	:		
		:	:		
		:	:		
		:	:		
		:	:		
		:	:		
		:	:		

NOTE:

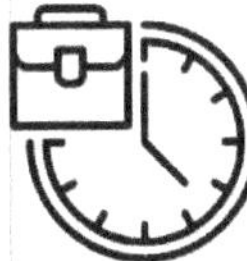 

WORK LOG

MONTH:

DATE	WORK ACTIVITY	START TIME	END TIME		TOTAL HOURS
		:	:		
		:	:		
		:	:		
		:	:		
		:	:		
		:	:		
		:	:		
		:	:		
		:	:		
		:	:		
		:	:		
		:	:		
		:	:		
		:	:		
		:	:		
		:	:		

NOTE: